Handbook
of the Clinical Treatment
# of Infidelity

Handbook of the Clinical Treatment of Infidelity has been co-published simultaneously as *Journal of Couple & Relationship Therapy*, Volume 4, Numbers 2/3 2005.

Monographic Separates from the *Journal of Couple & Relationship Therapy*™

For additional information on these and other Haworth Press titles, including descriptions, tables of contents, reviews, and prices, use the QuickSearch catalog at http://www.HaworthPress.com.

*The *Journal of Couple & Relationship Therapy* ™ is the successor title to *Journal of Couples Therapy* (Founding Editor: Barbara Jo Brothers, MSW), which changed title after Vol. 10, No. 3/4 2001. The journal is renumbered to start as Vol. 1, No. 1 2002.

Handbook of the Clinical Treatment of Infidelity, edited by Fred P. Piercy, PhD, Katherine M. Hertlein, PhD, and Joseph L. Wetchler, PhD (Vol. 4, No. 2/3, 2005). *"This book will be a useful addition to the libraries of marriage and family therapists as well as other clinicians who struggle to help their clients deal with their own or a partner's infidelities."*

Clinical Issues with Interracial Couples: Theories and Research, edited by Volker Thomas, PhD, Terri A. Karis, PhD, and Joseph L. Wetchler, PhD (Vol. 2, No. 2/3, 2003). *"A useful text in family systems and therapy courses. . . . A very useful, and even necessary, text for clinicians who do couples work and will increasingly be dealing with cross-cultural and interracial couples." (Maria P. P. Root, PhD, Psychologist, Seattle, Washington)*

Couples, Intimacy Issues, and Addiction, edited by Barbara Jo Brothers, MSW, BCD, CGP (Vol. 10, No. 3/4, 2001).* *"A much needed and insightful book for those who already work with couples, and a marvelous addition to the library of any new therapist just venturing into the field of couples therapy. This book opens windows to explore, with respect and understanding, the many ways of partnering." (Mary Ellen O'Hare-Lavin, PhD, Clinical Psychologist, Private Practice; Adjunct Faculty, Oakton Community College, Des Plaines, Illinois)*

Couples and Body Therapy, edited by Barbara Jo Brothers, MSW, BCD, CGP (Vol. 10, No. 2, 2001).* *"A wonderful revisiting and blending of two significant fields. Once digested, one wonders how the therapist can focus on the couple without addressing the bodies they inhabit." (Cindy Ashkins, PhD, LCSW, LMT, Couples Psychotherapist and Licensed Bodyworker in Private Practice, Metairie, North Carolina)*

The Abuse of Men: Trauma Begets Trauma, edited by Barbara Jo Brothers, MSW, BCSW (Vol. 10, No. 1, 2001).* *"Addresses a topic that has been neglected. . . . This book is unique in adopting a systematic perspective that focuses not solely on the males who have been abused but also on their partners and family members. . . . Gives detailed and specific directions for intervening with couples who have experienced multiple traumas." (Joseph A. Micucci, PhD, Associate Professor of Psychology, Chestnut Hill College, Pennsylvania)*

The Personhood of the Therapist, edited by Barbara Jo Brothers, MSW, BCSW (Vol. 9, No. 3/4, 2000).* *Through suggestions, techniques, examples, and case studies, this book will help you develop a great sense of openness about yourself and your feelings, enabling you to offer clients more effective services.*

Couples Connecting: Prerequisites of Intimacy, edited by Barbara Jo Brothers, MSW, BCSW (Vol. 9, No. 1/2, 2000).* *"Brothers views marriage as an ideal context for the psychological and spiritual evolution of human beings, and invites therapists to reflect on the role they can play in facilitating this. Readers are sure to recognize their clients among the examples given and to return to their work with a renewed vision of the possibilities for growth and change." (Eleanor D. Macklin, PhD, Emeritus Professor and former Director of the Marriage and Family Therapy program, Syracuse University, New York)*

Couples Therapy in Managed Care: Facing the Crisis, edited by Barbara Jo Brothers, MSW, BCSW (Vol. 8, No. 3/4, 1999).* *Provides social workers, psychologists, and counselors with an overview of the negative effects of the managed care industry on the quality of mental health care. Within this book, you will discover the paradoxes that occur with the mixing of business principles and service principles and find valuable suggestions on how you can creatively cope within the managed care context. With* Couples Therapy in Managed Care, *you will learn how you can remain true to your own integrity and still get paid for your work and offer quality services within the current context of managed care.*

Couples and Pregnancy: Welcome, Unwelcome, and In-Between, edited by Barbara Jo Brothers, MSW, BCSW (Vol. 8, No. 2, 1999).* *Gain valuable insight into how pregnancy and birth have a profound psychological effect on the parents' relationship, especially on their experience of intimacy.*

Couples, Trauma, and Catastrophes, edited by Barbara Jo Brothers, MSW, BCSW (Vol. 7, No. 4, 1998).* *Helps therapists and counselors working with couples facing major crises and trauma.*

Couples: A Medley of Models, edited by Barbara Jo Brothers, MSW, BCSW, BCD (Vol. 7, No. 2/3, 1998).* *"A wonderful set of authors who illuminate different corners of relationships. This book belongs on your shelf . . . but only after you've read it and loved it." (Derek Paar, PhD, Associate Professor of Psychology, Springfield College, Massachusetts)*

When One Partner Is Willing and the Other Is Not, edited by Barbara Jo Brothers, MSW, BCSW (Vol. 7, No. 1, 1997).* *"An engaging variety of insightful perspectives on resistance in couples therapy." (Stan Taubman, DSW, Director of Managed Care, Alameda County Behavioral Health Care Service, Berkeley, California; Author,* Ending the Struggle Against Yourself*)*

Couples and the Tao of Congruence, edited by Barbara Jo Brothers, MSW, BCSW (Vol. 6, No. 3/4, 1996).* *"A library of information linking Virginia Satir's teaching and practice of creative improvement in human relations and the Tao of Congruence. . . . A stimulating read." (Josephine A. Bates, DSW, BD, retired mental health researcher and family counselor, Lake Preston, South Dakota)*

Couples and Change, edited by Barbara Jo Brothers, MSW, BCSW (Vol. 6, No. 1/2, 1996).* *This enlightening book presents readers with Satir's observations–observations that show the difference between thinking with systems in mind and thinking linearly–of process, interrelatedness, and attitudes.*

Couples: Building Bridges, edited by Barbara Jo Brothers, MSW, BCSW (Vol. 5, No. 4, 1996).* *"This work should be included in the library of anyone considering to be a therapist or who is one or who is fascinated by the terminology and conceptualizations which the study of marriage utilizes." (Irv Loev, PhD, MSW-ACP, LPC, LMFT, private practitioner)*

Couples and Countertransference, edited by Barbara Jo Brothers, MSW, BCSW (Vol. 5, No. 3, 1995).* *"I would recommend this book to beginning and advanced couple therapists as well as to social workers and psychologists. . . . This book is a wealth of information." (International Transactional Analysis Association)*

Power and Partnering, edited by Barbara Jo Brothers, MSW, BCSW (Vol. 5, No. 1/2, 1995).* *"Appeals to therapists and lay people who find themselves drawn to the works of Virginia Satir and Carl Jung. Includes stories and research data satisfying the tastes of both left- and right-brained readers." (Virginia O. Felder, ThM, Licensed Marriage and Family Therapist, private practice, Atlanta, Georgia)*

Surpassing Threats and Rewards: Newer Plateaus for Couples and Coupling, edited by Barbara Jo Brothers, MSW, BCSW (Vol. 4, No. 3/4, 1995).* *Explores the dynamics of discord, rejection, and blame in the coupling process and provides practical information to help readers understand marital dissatisfaction and how this dissatisfaction manifests itself in relationships.*

Attraction and Attachment: Understanding Styles of Relationships, edited by Barbara Jo Brothers, MSW, BCSW (Vol. 4, No. 1/2, 1994).* *"Ideas on working effectively with couples. . . . I strongly recommend this book for those who want to have a better understanding of the complex dynamics of couples and couples therapy." (Gilbert J. Greene, PhD, ACSW, Associate Professor, College of Social Work, The Ohio State University)*

Peace, War, and Mental Health: Couples Therapists Look at the Dynamics, edited by Barbara Jo Brothers, MSW, BCSW (Vol. 3, No. 4, 1993).* *Discover how issues of world war and peace relate to the dynamics of couples therapy in this thought-provoking book.*

Handbook
of the Clinical Treatment
# of Infidelity

Fred P. Piercy, PhD
Katherine M. Hertlein, PhD
Joseph L. Wetchler, PhD
Editors

Handbook of the Clinical Treatment of Infidelity has been co-published simultaneously as *Journal of Couple & Relationship Therapy*, Volume 4, Numbers 2/3 2005.

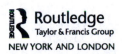

Routledge
Taylor & Francis Group
NEW YORK AND LONDON

First published by
The Haworth Press, Inc.
10 Alice Street
Binghamton, N Y 13904-1580

This edition published 2011 by Routledge

Routledge
Taylor & Francis Group
711 Third Avenue
New York, NY 10017

Routledge
Taylor & Francis Group
2 Park Square, Milton Park
Abingdon, Oxon OX14 4RN

Handbook of the Clinical Treatment of Infidelity has been co-published simultaneously as *Journal of Couple & Relationship Therapy*™, Volume 4 Numbers 2/3 2005.

The development, preparation, and publication of this work has been undertaken with great care. However, the publisher, employees, editors, and agents of The Haworth Press and all imprints of The Haworth Press, including The Haworth Medical Press® and Pharmaceutical Products Press®, are not responsible for any errors contained herein or for consequences that may ensue from use of materials or information contained in this work. Opinions expressed by the author(s) are not necessarily those of The Haworth Press. With regard to case studies, identities and circumstances of individuals discussed herein have been changed to protect confidentiality. Any resemblance to actual persons, living or dead, is entirely coincidental.

Cover design by Lora Wiggins

Library of Congress Cataloging-in-Publication Data

Handbook of the clinical treatment of infidelity / Fred P. Piercy, Katherine M. Hertlein, Joseph L. Wetchler, editors.
    p. cm.
    "Co-published simultaneously as Journal of couple & relationship therapy, Volume 4, numbers 2/3 2005."
    Includes bibliographical references and index.
    ISBN-10: 0-7890-2994-4 (hard cover : alk. paper)
    ISBN-13: 978-0-7890-2994-2(hard cover : alk. paper)
    ISBN-10: 0-7890-2995-2 (soft cover : alk. paper)
    ISBN 13: 978-0-7890-2995-9 (soft cover : alk. paper)
    1. Marital psychotherapy 2. Adultery–Treatment. I. Piercy, Fred P. II. Hertlein, Katherine M. III. Wetchler, Joseph L.
RC488.5.H335 2005
616.89'1562–dc22
                                          2005014002

Handbook of the Clinical Treatment of Infidelity

CONTENTS

ABOUT THE EDITORS

Fred P. Piercy, PhD, joined Virginia Tech in August, 2000, after 25 years of teaching family therapy, the last 18 of which were at Purdue University. Dr. Piercy received degrees from the University of Florida, University of South Carolina, and Wake Forest University. He is an active researcher, and has worked in a variety of mental health settings. Dr. Piercy has served two times on the Board of Directors of the American Association for Marriage and Family Therapy (AAMFT), and as the chair of the Commission on Accreditation for Marriage and Family Therapy Education. Dr. Piercy is also a member and Fellow in both AAMFT and the American Psychological Association.

Dr. Piercy's professional interests include family therapy education, family therapy for drug and alcohol abuse, qualitative research, hearing loss and couple communications, and social science HIV/AIDS prevention research and intervention. Dr. Piercy has written over 160 published articles, five books, and 35 funded grants. He is the co-editor of *Research Methods in Family Therapy* (2nd Edition) (with Douglas Sprenkle, Guilford Press, in press) and co-author of *Family Therapy Sourcebook* (with Douglas Sprenkle, Joseph Wetchler, and associates; Guilford Press, 1986, 1996) and *Stop Marital Fights Before They Start* (with Norman Lobsenz, Berkley Press, 1994). Dr. Piercy has won both national and university teaching awards. He has collaborated extensively with colleagues from the University of Indonesia and Atma Jaya University (in Jakarta, Indonesia) and was the principal investigator of a World AIDS Foundation funded project in Indonesia. Dr. Piercy has also consulted in Nepal, the Philippines, and India.

Katherine M. Hertlein, PhD, received her PhD in marriage and family therapy from Virginia Tech. She is Assistant Professor of Marriage and Family Therapy at the University of Nevada-Las Vegas. She has published in several journals including *Journal of Couple & Relationship Therapy, American Journal of Family Therapy, Contemporary Family Therapy, Journal of Feminist Family Therapy*, and *Journal of Clinical Activities, Assignments & Handouts in Psychotherapy Practice*. She serves as reviewer for several journals and as a co-editor for a book on therapy interventions for couples and families. Her areas of interest include research methodology and measurement, training in marriage and family therapy, and infidelity treatment.

Joseph L. Wetchler, PhD, is Professor and Director of the Marriage and Family Therapy Program at Purdue University Calumet, Hammond, Indiana. He is a Clinical Member and Approved Supervisor of the American Association for Marriage and Family Therapy. Dr. Wetchler was the recipient of the 2004 Purdue University Calumet Outstanding Faculty Scholar Award and 1997 Indiana Association for Marriage and Family Therapy Award for Outstanding Contribution to Research in Family Life. He has served on the Editoral Boards of the *American Journal of Family Therapy,* the *Journal of Feminist Family Therapy,* the *Journal of GLBT Family Studies,* the *Journal of Marital and Family Therapy,* and the *Journal of Clinical Activities, Assignments & Handouts in Psychotherapy Practice.* Dr. Wetchler is a co-editor (with Jerry Bigner) of *Relationship Therapy with Same-Sex Couples*, a co-editor (with Volker Thomas and Terri Karis) of *Clinical Issues with Interracial Couples*, co-editor (with Lorna Hecker) of *An Introduction to Marriage and Family Therapy* and a co-author (with Fred Piercy and Douglas Sprenkle) of the *Family Therapy Sourcebook, 2nd edition.* He is also the author of numerous journal articles on family therapy supervision, family therapy for child and adolescent problems, couple therapy for substance abuse, and the self of the therapist. Dr. Wetchler has been a co-investigator on a large project funded by the National Institute on Drug Abuse to study couple therapy approaches for substance-abusing women. He regularly consults to social service agencies and therapists in private practice, and maintains an active couple and family therapy practice in Northwest Indiana. Dr. Wetchler is a licensed marriage and family therapist in Indiana.

Acknowledgments

We are so grateful to all of the contributors who, through their insight and dedication to couples, have helped make this volume a reality. Further, we want to thank the editors and staff at The Haworth Press, Inc. for their enormous support of this project. Finally, we would like to thank our families for all of their love and support:

(FP) Thanks to Susan, for all the usual reasons, and many, many more.

(KH) This volume would not have been possible without the encouragement and support of my husband, Eric. Further, I wish to dedicate this book to my sisters, Denise, Anne, and Lynn, for the years of support, joy, and laughter.

(JW) Thanks to Jessica Lily, Jessica Marie, and Ryan for keeping me young, and special thanks to my wife, Carole, who initially approached me with the idea for this book. I love all of you!

Fred P. Piercy
Katherine M. Hertlein
Joseph L. Wetchler

Introduction

In the film *Love Actually*, a middle-aged Emma Thompson finds her Christmas present in her husband's coat pocket–a beautiful necklace. She smiles and thinks, "He bought me something romantic." The scene cuts to Christmas morning, and Emma opens the box with her necklace, only to find a CD of singer Joni Mitchell instead. In that instant Emma knows that the necklace was meant for another woman. We see her confusion, hurt, anger. She puts on a cheery front for her children, though, as they open their gifts. We hear Joni Mitchell's song in the background:

> I've looked at love from both sides now,
> From give and take,
> And still somehow,
> It's love's illusions I recall,
> I really don't know love at all. . .

Affairs disorient, and love seems less real in the wake of betrayal. As couple therapists, we have seen Emma's pain in the eyes of our clients. Affairs bring an inside-out devastation to relationships that words can't capture.

How can we help our clients survive infidelity? That's the focus of this book. We have brought together an impressive group of experts to reflect on issues central to affairs, and how to help couples heal and learn from them. The authors address the subject with freshness and insight, sometimes from different theoretical orientations, but always with humanity and seasoned wisdom.

Susan Johnson, the co-developer of Emotionally Focused Therapy (EFT), discusses affairs through the lens of attachment theory. She sees

[Haworth co-indexing entry note]: "Introduction." Piercy, Fred P., Katherine M. Hertlein, and Joseph L. Wetchler. Co-published simultaneously in *Journal of Couple & Relationship Therapy* (The Haworth Press) Vol. 4, No. 2/3, 2005, pp. 1-3; and: *Handbook of the Clinical Treatment of Infidelity* (ed: Fred P. Piercy, Katherine M. Hertlein, and Joseph L. Wetchler) The Haworth Press, Inc., 2005, pp. 1-3. Single or multiple copies of this article are available for a fee from The Haworth Document Delivery Service [1-800-HAWORTH, 9:00 a.m. - 5:00 p.m. (EST). E-mail address: docdelivery@haworthpress.com].

Available online at http://www.haworthpress.com/web/JCRT
doi:10.1300/J398v04n02_01

infidelity as a violation of trust that ruptures the attachment bond between partners. EFT, Johnson contends, provides a way to acknowledge and express pain, remorse, and regret, and to repair this attachment bond.

David Moultrup believes that there are no easy answers. Therapy for him is the process of informed exploration (sometimes intergenerational, sometimes interpersonal) that can help couples learn and grow from an affair.

Frank Pittman and Tina Pittman Wagers outline cultural myths about affairs (e.g., "This marriage was a mistake."), and do their share of debunking. They say, for example, that "those who expect marriage to make them happy are missing the point. Marriage is not supposed to make people happy; it is supposed to make people married. . ." Happiness, they contend, is a choice, and if people want to feel more in love, they should act more loving.

Other authors emphasize certain aspects of infidelity treatment that, for them, are integral to the process of healing. Adrian Blow discusses how to help couples address their pain, and the healing process, head-on. Brian Case highlights the role of apology and forgiveness in this process. Frank Stalfa and Catherine Hastings focus on the treatment of "accusatory suffering"–a spouse's obsessive holding onto and retaliating for the affair long after the affair has ended, and despite the offending partner's repeated apologies and efforts at restitution. Don-David Lusterman discusses partners who have suppressed or denied traumatic stress reactions (analogous to "cold rage") to their partner's affair, and how to help them.

Scott Johnson discusses "nonsense" about affairs, from who is cheatin' on whom, to whether men really have more affairs than women, to the blame-filled language of "affairs" and "betrayal" and "infidelity." Johnson asks us to think more systemically about affairs, and to see the dynamics of extradyadic relationships as more complex and nuanced than they are typically portrayed in the literature.

With the advent of the Internet, people who want to be unfaithful have an inexpensive, legal, accessible, anonymous vehicle to do so. Consequently, Internet infidelity has become a cottage industry. Joan Atwood provides an overview of Internet infidelity, the factors influencing one's involvement in this type of infidelity, and some of the considerations for therapists. Tim Nelson, Fred Piercy, and Doug Sprenkle report on the results of a multi-phase Delphi study that explored what infidelity experts say are the critical issues, interventions, and gender differences in the treatment of Internet infidelity. Monica Whitty and Adrian Carr draw from Klein's object relations theory and discuss how this might influence how people might rationalize their Internet infidelity.

Emily Brown outlines the concept of the Split Self Affair. She discusses its origins, its characteristics, and implications for the individuals and the couples. Further, she provides detailed information on how to work with these couples in therapy.

Michael Bettinger presents extra dyadic relationships as a fact, rather than a problem, for many gay male relationships. He discusses gay male polyamory as an alternative to the heterosexual model of emotional and sexual exclusivity in romantic dyadic relationships, and provides a role for therapists to help certain gay male couples develop rules around the inclusion of outside partners.

Finally, Katherine Hertlein and Gary Skaggs report on the results of a study that assessed the level of differentiation and one's engagement in extra dyadic relationships. They found that level of differentiation and participation in affairs were not significantly related among the subjects in their sample. This runs counter to what some have theorized and what some studies have found.

So, in this collection of papers our authors, to paraphrase Joni Mitchell, look at love (and infidelity) from many sides. Their cumulative wisdom should help couple therapists treat this difficult, but all-to-common presenting problem. We thank them for helping us help others face the challenges of infidelity.

Fred P. Piercy, PhD
Katherine M. Hertlein, PhD
Joseph L. Wetchler, PhD

Infidelity:
An Overview

Katherine M. Hertlein
Joseph L. Wetchler
Fred P. Piercy

SUMMARY. In this article, we provide an overview of infidelity theory, research, and treatment. We discuss the effect of infidelity on couples and delineate three types of infidelity–emotional, physical, and infidelity including aspects of both. Further, we expand traditional thinking about infidelity by reviewing the role of the Internet in infidelity, and explore infidelity within the context of comarital relationships. Finally, we discuss the overarching theories and common models used in infidelity treatment. *[Article copies available for a fee from The Haworth Document Delivery Service: 1-800-HAWORTH. E-mail address: <docdelivery@ haworthpress.com> Website: <http://www.HaworthPress.com> © 2005 by The Haworth Press, Inc. All rights reserved.]*

KEYWORDS. Infidelity, extramarital, affairs, treatment, couples

Katherine M. Hertlein, PhD, is Adjunct Faculty, Marriage and Family Therapy Program at Virginia Tech, 840 University City Boulevard, Suite 1, Blacksburg, VA 24061.
Joseph L. Wetchler, PhD, is Professor and Director, Marriage and Family Therapy Program, Purdue University Calumet, Hammond, IN 46323.
Fred P. Piercy, PhD, is Department Head of Human Development, Virginia Tech, 366 Wallace Hall, Blacksburg, VA 24601.

[Haworth co-indexing entry note]: "Infidelity: An Overview." Hertlein, Katherine M., Joseph L. Wetchler, and Fred P. Piercy. Co-published simultaneously in *Journal of Couple & Relationship Therapy* (The Haworth Press) Vol. 4, No. 2/3, 2005, pp. 5-16; and: *Handbook of the Clinical Treatment of Infidelity* (ed: Fred P. Piercy, Katherine M. Hertlein, and Joseph L. Wetchler) The Haworth Press, Inc., 2005, pp. 5-16. Single or multiple copies of this article are available for a fee from The Haworth Document Delivery Service [1-800-HAWORTH, 9:00 a.m. - 5:00 p.m. (EST). E-mail address: docdelivery@haworthpress.com].

Available online at http://www.haworthpress.com/web/JCRT
© 2005 by The Haworth Press, Inc. All rights reserved.
doi:10.1300/J398v04n02_02

Unfaithful spouses have been around a long time, leaving havoc in their wake. Infidelity is a major reason for marital dissolution (Brown, 1999; Pittman, 1989) and provided as the primary presenting problem during the course of couple therapy (Subotnik & Harris, 1999). Infidelity can impair the trust, connection, and intimacy level within couples. Partners often find it difficult to trust one another or to recover from the pain and loss. They may need to decide whether they will move forward with their relationship or individually. Because of the emotions experienced by the couple, decisions made during the crisis, and the delicacy of managing their relationship after the crisis, practitioners who work with couples and families need to be able to understand and address the unique treatment issues of infidelity (Atkins, Baucom, & Jacobson, 2001; Whisman, Dixon, & Johnson, 1997).

DEFINITIONS AND FREQUENCY OF INFIDELITY

Historically, infidelity was considered the breaking of a contract of sexual exclusivity between two people who are dating, married, or otherwise in a committed relationship. Yet, more recently, the definition has expanded to include a wide range of behaviors. For some, part of the definition of infidelity includes participation in sexual intercourse with a person other than one's partner. Others include behaviors such as cybersex (or sex over the computer using words), viewing pornography, varying degrees of physical intimacy, such as kissing and holding hands, and even emotional intimacy with another person to the detriment of the primary relationship.

At its very core, infidelity refers to any behavior that breaks the contract that two people have with each other (Lusterman, 1998). What is especially complex about the broad definition of infidelity is that two different people in the same relationship might have different ideas about what represents infidelity or constitutes an affair. Thus, the problems related to infidelity may stretch beyond the impact of the events themselves, often forcing couples to revisit their relationship contract. Other issues caused by infidelity are those related to the time, energy, and resources spent to maintain another relationship.

The percentage of people engaging in infidelity is estimated anywhere from 15% to 70% (Hite, 1987; Johnson, 1972; Kinsey, Pomeroy, & Martin, 1948; Kinsey, Pomeroy, Martin, & Gebhard, 1953; Wyatt, Peters, & Guthrie, 1988a; 1988b). Kinsey and his colleagues performed one of the first inclusive studies on human sexual behavior

(Bullough, 1998; Kim, 1969; Kinsey et al., 1948; Kinsey et al., 1953) and found approximately 30% of the population surveyed had engaged in extramarital coitus at least once in their lives (between 23% and 37% of men and approximately 30% of women). Hite (1987, 1984) reported that 70% of women seek sex outside of their marriage after four to five years as compared to 72% of men after two years of marriage. Other estimates suggest the number for both males and females may be lower (Nass, Libby, & Fisher, 1981), between 45% to 55% of the population. In 1996, 369 people (both men and women) responding to the General Social Survey admitted to engaging in sex with someone other than their marital partner, and 1,618 stated they did not, for a percentage of 18.5% (GSS, 1999). This percentage demonstrates an increase over the previous five years (14.6%). Finally, Laumann, Gagnon, Michaels, and Michael (1994), found that number to be between 11% and 24% for men and women.

Infidelity is not only restricted to the marital relationship, but is also considered a problem in dating relationships (Drigotas, Safstrom, & Gentilia, 1999; Hansen, 1987; Lieberman, 1988), impacting as many as 30% of dating couples (Sheppard, Nelson, & Andreoli-Mathie, 1995). Some suggest that infidelity in dating will carry over into the marriage (Drigotas, Safstrom, & Gentilia, 1999); however, even if infidelity does not carry over into a marital relationship, most couples (cohabitating or married) exhibit similar behavior patterns (Thompson, 1984). Hansen (1987) found men and women with more dating experience are more likely to have affairs, and reports about 71% of men and 57% of women in dating relationships have engaged in an extradyadic relationship at some point in their dating history.

EFFECTS OF INFIDELITY

Infidelity has a significant impact on couples and families. Its effects can flow though the couple as well as affect family relationships and a couple's social support network (Subotnik & Harris, 1999). There are psychological impacts for both those having the affair and for their partners. After the revelation of an affair, a couple may have to decide whether to stay together (Subotnik & Harris, 1999; Vaughan, 2003). Those whose partners have had affairs feel a sense of betrayal and anger at their partner. They may also feel angry with themselves for "missing the signs," or not being there for their loved one. Added to this may be a sense of embarrassment and shame about these events (Vaughan,

2003). Also, the uninvolved partners may lose trust in their partner, and feel betrayed (Spring, 1996; Vaughan, 2003). They may also feel a loss of identity, sense of specialness with their partner, and sense of purpose (Spring, 1996). The betrayed partner may incessantly inquire about their partner's activities, wonder if they are where they say they are, or whether they are secretly meeting with the third party. Because of the continual inquiries and the attempts of the involved partner to justify his/her behavior, a hierarchy may be established within the relationship: in other words, the involved partner may feel pressure to report on his/her activities to the partner, with the uninvolved partner passing judgment on the other's actions. This hierarchy can cause further problems for the couple and have implications for the balance of power within the relationship.

For the person who becomes involved with a third party, some of the psychological effects might include guilt and loss of self-esteem. The person might also feel the need to protect his/her partner from hurt related to the infidelity. This guilt and need to protect may prevent the person from talking with the partner about the affair, and may hinder the extent to which such couples can process their feelings and work on their relationship (Vaughan, 2003). For both partners, there may also potentially be some fear. The revelation of an affair puts the couple in a position where, if they decide to work on the relationship, they will have to confront some difficult issues. In an environment where there has been a betrayal of trust, such as in cases of infidelity, it becomes difficult for couples to feel safe enough to communicate with one another. This further exacerbates those issues behind the infidelity, and increases the difficulty of resolving them.

Finally, infidelity may exact a physical toll. The chronic stress, agitation, and exhaustion of dealing with this issue may lead to health problems for both partners. Added to this stress, there is also the potential threat of the involved partner introducing sexually transmitted diseases into the primary relationship. Some, such as HIV and herpes, can be lifelong conditions, significantly affecting the life of each partner and their families.

TYPES OF INFIDELITY

The literature describes different types of infidelity: physical, emotional, and infidelity that combines elements of both. Physical and emotional infidelities not only differ in what characterizes them, but also in their effects on the primary relationship. Infidelity, as most people conceive it, refers to a sexual relationship with a third person. Thompson (1984) defines an affair as "genital sexual involvement outside the marriage without the express knowledge or consent of one's partner" (p. 36). Some authors and researchers use it interchangeably with the terms "extramarital sex" or "extramarital coitus" (Bell, Turner, & Rosen, 1975; Thompson, 1983). Behaviors other than intercourse that might characterize physical infidelity include kissing, petting, and/or sexual interactions other than intercourse (Roscoe, Cavanaugh, & Kennedy, 1988; Yarab, Sensibaugh, & Allgeier, 1998).

Emotional Infidelity

Emotional infidelity, rather than being characterized by a physical component, is instead defined by emotional intimacy and connection shared by two people to the exclusion of one of their partners (Collins, 1999; Drigotas, Safstrom, & Gentilia, 1999; Shackelford, 1997; Spring, 1996). An emotional affair occurs when one invests resources such as romantic love, time, and attention in another person other than the partner (Shackelford, 1997). Aspects of emotional intimacy may include sharing, understanding, companionship, self-esteem, and an otherwise close relationship (Glass & Wright, 1992). Moultrup (1990) refers to infidelity as an emotional solution to an emotional problem. Emotional affairs also appear to be more prevalent than physical affairs. Glass (2003), for example, reports that 44% of husbands and 57% of wives in her study indicated that in their affair, they had a strong emotional involvement to the other person without intercourse. Further, women are more likely to have an emotional component in their infidelity than men (Glass & Wright, 1985; Shackelford, 1997; Sheppard, Nelson, & Andreoli-Mathie, 1995). Emotional intimacy is clearly a powerful bond maintaining an affair (Glass, 2003).

Internet Infidelity

Online romances, though they may involve sexual behaviors, have more in common with emotional infidelity because they are characterized by emotional connection, rather than judgments on physical attractiveness or physical sexuality (Cooper & Sportlotari, 1997). One survey found that 75% of adults in the United States report they use email to flirt with someone to whom they are attracted ("The Email Dating

Game," 2001). Cooper, Scherer, and Mathy (2001) found approximately 20% of all Internet users report engaging in some sexual activity online. Further, as many as 26.3% of Internet users stated they have established at least one romantic interpersonal relationship with someone online (Parks & Roberts, 1996).

Cooper (2002) developed the "triple A" engine model which delineates three aspects unique to Internet infidelity: accessibility, affordability, and anonymity. Accessibility refers to the access an individual has to the Internet. Individuals most likely to engage in online infidelity are those with easy access to the Internet. Affordability refers to the cost of engaging in Internet infidelity. Cooper (2002) asserts that the principle of affordability works on the concept of supply and demand. For a very small price, a computer user can visit a multiple number of sites and get multiple sexual needs met. Additionally, people who might feel uncomfortable purchasing sexually charged material in stores can quickly download similar information in the privacy of their own home. Finally, anonymity refers to the ability of promoting any identity on the Internet one would like (Cooper, 2002). In person, carrying on an affair means the other person gets to know who you are, can see you, and can potentially judge you. On the Internet, users can backspace, erase, and change what they say in order to promote a specific identity.

Similarly, Leiblum, and Döring (2002) proposed a "triple C" engine which focuses on the interactive component of the Internet. "Communication" refers to the messages sent back and forth between respondents. "Collaboration" refers to the interaction between two respondents online. Finally, "Communities online" also provide another forum for interaction. These communities may refer to places online where people can gather and chat, generating a virtual social group within the confines of one's computer.

OPEN MARRIAGE, SWINGERS, AND POLYAMOROUS RELATIONSHIPS

Some couples may not find extradyadic sexual relationships to be problematic, and, in some cases, find them to be enhancing of their primary relationship. Three examples are found among couples involved in open marriages, couples involved in a swingers lifestyle, and some gay males and lesbian females involved in polyamorous relationships.

Open Marriage

Open marriage involves a willingness by both members of a couple to engage in sexual relationships outside of the primary dyad. In an early study of couples involved in open marriage, Knapp (1976) found that the majority of respondents believed that the outside sexual involvement enhanced fulfillment of their personal needs, increased sexual satisfaction within their marriage, increased communication with their spouse, and lessened jealousy and possessiveness. Still, some of the participants expressed problems with jealousy, guilt, and time-sharing problems. Interestingly enough, the majority of respondents in her sample felt "the advantages of co-marital sex significantly outweighed the disadvantages" (Knapp, 1976, p. 214). Further, in the majority of these couples a major component of their marriage involved the honesty of both partners about their outside relationships. Finally, in a five-year follow-up of couples in sexually open marriages (Rubin & Adams, 1986), the majority of couples were still married, though not as many as the control sample of sexually exclusive couples. Also, there were no significant differences in marital satisfaction between these groups.

Swinger Lifestyle

Couples involved in a swinger lifestyle jointly share partners with other couples, or in groups, solely for sexual purposes (Buunk & van Driel, 1989). This group appears to comprise 1 to 2% of the population, although the studies are dated (e.g., Bartell, 1971; Cole & Spaniard, 1974; Hunt, 1974). Further, it appears that the majority of couples engage in swinging activities only once (Jenks, 1998). As with open marriage, many swingers report that swinging has a positive effect on their marriage (Jenks, 1998; Levitt, 1988; Varni, 1974). Still, some state that swinging negatively impacted their relationship (Levitt, 1988). Jenks (1998) reports that a primary factor among swingers is that the sharing of partners is open and maintained on a purely sexual level. Hidden relationships and the addition of emotional involvement may lead to problems in the primary relationship. While positive outcomes have been reported by couples in open marriages and swinging relationships, these types of relationships are not necessarily models for most couples. They are practiced by a minority of couples and the reported enhancement to their relationships may be due to factors separate from their sexual behavior.

Polyamorous Relationships Among Gay Men and Lesbian Women

Polyamory, or the sexual and emotional involvement with more than one partner, is practiced among some members of the gay (Anapol, 1997; Bettinger, 2005) and lesbian (Hall, 2004; Munson and Stellborn, 1999) communities. Polyamorous relationships can range from a primary dyad with one or more secondary partners to a situation in which three or more individuals share a primary sexual and emotional relationship with each other (Bettinger, 2005). Bettinger (2004) states that it is helpful to separate emotional and sexual monogamy when working with gay male couples. While some gay male couples may discuss whether or not to have outside sexual relationships, others may have to negotiate the rules around when and where outside sexual partners are permissible. Unfortunately, most research on mating patterns and relationship satisfaction have been conducted on heterosexual couples. Thus, research is necessary on these same phenomena within the gay and lesbian communities (Bettinger, 2005).

INFIDELITY TREATMENT

There are several common factors in infidelity treatment that cut across theoretical orientations. One such common factor is manipulating the environment. One part of conventional infidelity treatment involves discontinuing the affair during the relationship. Elbaum (1981), for example, indicates that therapists should ask the involved spouse to break off the extradyadic relationship for the duration of treatment. Environmental strategies in cases of Internet infidelity might include moving the computer to another room, using a program to restrict visits to specific sites, or limiting time on the computer.

Several infidelity treatment models have similar assessment components in common. Similar to most couple cases, the first component in the assessment includes taking an adequate couple history (Lusterman, 1998). A second component includes assessing and understanding the context of the affair within the primary relationship (e.g., Gordon & Baucom, 1999). Westfall (1989) suggests that therapists identify the extent of the infidelity in terms of the extent of secrecy and the involvement with the other person. Pittman and Wagers (1995) also suggest that therapists determine what type of affair occurred (e.g., an ongoing relationship or a one-time event). Weeks and Treat (2001) outline specific important considerations in the assessment of infidelity. These include exploring: (a) the duration of the affair, (b) number of sexual partners, (c) gender of the third party, (d) level of sexual activity, (e) whether each partner was having an affair, (f) degree of emotional involvement or attachment, (g) each person's relationship to the third party, (h) extent of lies and secrecy around the affair, (i) degree to which the other person knew about or consented to the affair, and (j) the tolerance of the affair by the social network of the person or couple.

Another factor common to many models and strategies is goal setting. An important goal for couples facing infidelity issues is whether they want to continue their relationship (Lusterman, 1998; Spring, 1996). An answer to this question would determine the course of therapy. Of course, this goal could change depending on how the course of treatment progresses. For those couples electing to stay together these goals might include shifting focus and rebuilding trust (Guerin, Fay, Burden, & Kautto, 1987). Such strategies to meet this would be improving couple communication skills, developing trust, and encouraging the couple to be honest with one another (Elbaum, 1981).

While therapists use common strategies for use in infidelity treatment, they use a range of theories to guide their treatment. These include transgenerational theories, emotionally-focused therapies, solution-focused therapies, and other relationally-based theories. Bowen systems theory underlies Moultrup's (1990) treatment of infidelity. Moultrup (1990) has identified several multigenerational aspects to infidelity. For example, he contends that some couples have patterns of infidelity existing within several generations of their family and that infidelity may be related to one's level of differentiation. Other clinicians and researchers see infidelity as an example of triangulation (e.g., Moultrup, 1990; Lusterman, 1998; Spring, 1996). Based on Bowen systems theory (1978), Pittman and Wagers (1995) suggest that therapists also need to manage a couple's anxiety in the room by providing a safe environment. Only after an assessment of the issues at hand and an ability to manage anxiety and emotional reactivity, can a post-affair couple find solutions to their problems.

Emotionally-focused therapy (Greenberg & Johnson, 1988) guides the work of a growing number of family therapists. One large piece of emotionally focused work is promoting safety and security in the therapy room. Glass (2002) sees her treatment as akin to PTSD treatment. Within this framework, the therapist is encouraged to promote an environment of safety and hope for the couple. In this environment, the couple can come together and share their story.

Lusterman (1998), who holds to a largely eclectic theoretical framework, helps couples to develop trust and honesty with each other as part of his treatment. Further, he helps couples to identify how to deal with the anger and the hurt caused by the infidelity in a productive manner.

Many therapists incorporate aspects of solution-focused theory base in infidelity work. Pittman and Wagers (1995), for example, seek to identify what couples need to move forward from the infidelity. They encourage therapists to, after addressing the emotional reactivity, find solutions and to implement these solutions in their treatment. For example, therapists may work with couples to identify what things were working for them in the relationship prior to the affair, how they meet one another's needs, and increase these behaviors in the relationship.

There are certainly other relationally based frameworks that a therapist may use to guide his or her work with infidelity cases. For example, Westfall (1989) works with therapists to connect the infidelity events to larger problems within the relationship. Many therapists also encourage the couple to work on communication strategies related to the affair (e.g., Lusterman, 1998), such as discussing the pain and hurt and using communication so that each person understands one another's needs (Subotnik & Harris, 1999; Vaughan, 2003).

CONCLUSION

The problem of treating infidelity is a thorny one for clinicians. With numerous definitions, types, relationship outcome decisions, and even questions regarding whether or not extramarital infidelity is a problem for some couples, it is no wonder that many couple therapists are at a loss for how to proceed with treatment. While some common factors exist across treatments, perhaps the most important components when treating infidelity are an open mind and clinical flexibility. We hope that this volume will broaden both the way you see infidelity and how you help couples survive and (in time) thrive in its wake.

REFERENCES

Anapol, D. (1997). *Polyamory: The new love without limits.* San Rafael, CA: IntiNet Resource Center.

Atkins, D. C., Baucom, D. H., & Jacobson, N. S. (2001). Understanding infidelity: Correlates in a national random sample. *Journal of Family Psychology, 15*(4), 735-749.

Hertlein, Wetchler, and Piercy

Bartell, G. D. (1971). *Group sex.* New York: Wyden.

Bettinger, M. (2005). Polyamory and gay men: A family systems approach. *Journal of GLBT Family Studies, 1,* 97-116.

Bettinger, M. (2004). A systems approach to sex therapy with gay male couples. *Journal of Couple & Relationship Therapy, 3* (2/3), 65-74.

Bowen, M. (1978). *Family therapy in clinical practice.* New York: Jason Aronson.

Brown, E. M. (1999). *Affairs: A guide to working through the repercussions of infidelity.* San Francisco, CA: Jossey-Bass.

Buunk, B. P., & van Driel, B. (1989). *Alternative lifestyles and relationships.* Newbury Park, CA: Sage.

Cole, C. L., & Spaniard, G. B. (1974). Comarital mate-sharing and family stability. *The Journal of Sex Research, 10,* 21-31.

Drigotas, S. M., Safstrom, C. A., & Gentilia, T. (1999). An investment model prediction of dating infidelity. *Journal of Personality and Social Psychology, 77*(3), 509-524.

Greenberg, L., & Johnson, S. (1988). *Emotionally focused therapy for couples.* New York: Guilford.

Hall, M. (2004). Resolving the curious paradox of the (a) sexual lesbian. *Journal of Couple & Relationship Therapy, 3*(2/3), 75-84.

Hansen, G. L. (1987). Extradyadic relations during courtship. *Journal of Sex Research, 23,* 382-390.

Hatala, M. N., Milewski, K., & Baack, D. W. (1999). Downloading love: A content analysis of Internet personal ads placed by college students. *College Student Journal, 33*(1), 124-129.

Hunt, M. (1974). *Sexual behavior in the 1970s.* Chicago: Dell.

Jenks, R. J. (1998). Swinging: A review of the literature. *Archives of Sexual Behavior, 27,* 507-520.

Knapp, J. (1976). An exploratory study of seventeen sexually open marriages. *The Journal of Sex Research, 12,* 206-219.

Laumann, E. O., Gagnon, J. H., Michael, R. T., & Michaels, S. (1994). *The social organization of sexuality: Sexual practices in the United States.* Chicago: University of Chicago Press.

Leiblum, S., & Döring, N. (2002). Internet sexuality: Known risks and fresh chances for women. In A. Cooper (Ed.), *Sex and the Internet: A guidebook for clinicians.* New York: Brunner-Routledge.

Levitt, E. E. (1988). Alternative life style and marital satisfaction: A brief report. *Annals of Sex Research, 1,* 455-461.

Lieberman, B. (1988). Extrapremarital intercourse: Attitudes towards a neglected sexual behavior. *Journal of Sex Research, 24,* 291-299.

Lieblum, S. R. (1997). Sex and the net: Clinical implications. *Journal of Sex Education and Therapy, 22*(1), 21-27.

Lusterman, D. (1998). *Infidelity: A survival guide.* New York: MJF Books.

Munson, M., & Stelbourn, J. (Eds.). (1999). *The lesbian polyamory reader.* Albany, NY: Harrington Park Press.

Pittman, F. (1989). *Private lies.* New York: W. W. Norton & Co.

Rubin, A. M., & Adams, J. R. (1986). Outcomes of sexually open marriages. *The Journal of Sex Research, 22,* 311-319

Spring, J. A. (1996). *After the affair: Healing the pain and rebuilding the trust when a partner has been unfaithful.* New York: Harper Collins.

Subotnik, R., & Harris, G. G. (1999). *Surviving infidelity (2nd ed.).* Avon, MA: Adams Media Corporation.

"The Email Dating Game." (2001). The email dating game. (2001, February 12). Retrieved November 22, 2001, from http://www.emarketer.com/estatnews/email_marketing/20010212_email_flirt.html

Varni, C. A. (1974). An exploratory study of spouse swapping. In J.R. Smith & L.G. Smith (Eds.), *Beyond monogamy: Recent studies on sexual alternatives in marriage.* Baltimore: Johns Hopkins Press.

Vaughan, P. (2003). *The monogamy myth.* New York: New Market Press.

CLINICAL MODELS

Broken Bonds:
An Emotionally Focused Approach to Infidelity

Susan M. Johnson

SUMMARY. Infidelity comes in many forms. Different meanings may be assigned to the various forms. This article discusses not only the different forms infidelity may take, but also the larger issue in the field of couple and family therapy; the meaning frame for understanding the impact of different kinds of events, specific relationship problems, and how to deal with them. This is done through the use of emotion focused therapy and the context of adult attachment. *[Article copies available for a fee from The Haworth Document Delivery Service: 1-800-HAWORTH. E-mail address: <docdelivery@ haworthpress.com> Website: <http://www.HaworthPress.com> © 2005 by The Haworth Press, Inc. All rights reserved.]*

Susan M. Johnson, EdD, is Professor of Psychology, University of Ottawa, and Director of Ottawa Couple and Family Institute, OCFI #201, 1869 Carling Avenue, Ottawa, Canada K2A 1E6.

[Haworth co-indexing entry note]: "Broken Bonds: An Emotionally Focused Approach to Infidelity." Johnson, Susan M. Co-published simultaneously in *Journal of Couple & Relationship Therapy* (The Haworth Press) Vol. 4, No. 2/3, 2005, pp. 17-29; and: *Handbook of the Clinical Treatment of Infidelity* (ed: Fred P. Piercy, Katherine M. Hertlein, and Joseph L. Wetchler) The Haworth Press, Inc., 2005, pp. 17-29. Single or multiple copies of this article are available for a fee from The Haworth Document Delivery Service [1-800-HAWORTH, 9:00 a.m. - 5:00 p.m. (EST). E-mail address: docdelivery@haworthpress.com].

KEYWORDS. Infidelity, attachment, emotionally focused couples therapy, forgiveness

Infidelity comes in all shapes and sizes. A one night stand at a professional conference that is framed as a superficial chance encounter or a four-year alternate relationship that involves day-to-day deception and strong emotional involvement. Some people begin an affair in order to end a marriage; some people state that they believe their marriage is fine and they also want to have an occasional "recreational" affair. Infidelity also can be interpreted in many different ways. One spouse may be able to accept a partner briefly turning to another in particular circumstances, another spouse may not be able to tolerate even a flirtation that does not result in actual intercourse, or finding photos of a scantily clad secretary in her husband's briefcase. Sex and sex with people other than your spouse has different meanings for different people. However, in general, perceived infidelity is experienced as a threat to adult love relationships and undermines the stability of these relationships. It is almost as damaging to these relationships as physical abuse (Whisman, Dixon, & Johnson, 1997) and it is a frequent precursor to seeking couple therapy.

The issue of the host of different meanings that can be assigned to infidelity echoes a larger issue in the field of couple and family therapy, namely the lack of a coherent well-researched theory of adult love to serve as a context–a meaning frame for understanding the impact of different kinds of events, specific relationship problems and how to deal with them. The Emotionally Focused model (Greenberg & Johnson, 1988; Johnson, 1996; Johnson, 2002) views adult love relationships through the lens of attachment theory (Bowlby, 1969, 1988; Johnson, 2003 a, b). Infidelity is then seen as a potentially devastating threat to attachment security that hyper-activates the deceived spouse's attachment needs and fears and so creates a crisis that must be addressed and resolved if the relationship is to survive and thrive. This chapter will discuss infidelity–defined in the dictionary as unfaithfulness–in terms of attachment theory and as a potential attachment injury (Johnson, Makinen, & Millikin, 2001) that undermines the attachment bond between partners.

When an EFT therapist listens to spouses describe the impact of their partners extra-marital involvement with another, he/she hears that these clients talk in attachment terms. In my office, Margie told her husband, "What hurts the most is that *I was not in your mind–I did not matter to you* in these moments with her. You did not *take me into account.* You were willing to risk our relationship for this 'excitement.' *How can I ever depend on you again*? Also, you lied to me and broke our commitment. I am wounded–I have *lost the sense of us* as a couple. And when I asked you–when I was weeping and asking you–you avoided, shrugged it off–like *my pain didn't matter to you* and you tried to put me off and cajole me with hugs. I can't hug you–let you close. I can't kiss you–thinking that you gave her kisses too. But I *can't bear the distance between us* either. I *need your reassurance*–and I don't believe it if you give it. There is *no safety–no ground to stand on* here." These words (especially those italicized) echo the observations of attachment theorists who point out that a secure attachment is based on a sense that you exist and are prized in the mind of the other, that you can depend on the other when you need him/her and that this other will cherish and protect rather than reject or abandon you. When this sense is shattered there is a traumatic loss and the process of separation distress, angry protest alternating with seeking contact and clinging to the other, as well as depression and despair are elicited. Margie's final words about her ambivalence, her distancing and her need, also echo the words of theorists who point out that attachment dilemmas where the loved one is both the source of and solution to pain are fundamentally disorganizing and overwhelming to deal with. For many clients, affairs constitute what EFT therapists have termed an attachment injury (Johnson, 2002), a trauma or wound, a violation of trust that brings the nature of the whole relationship into question and must be dealt with if the relationship is to survive. This paper will explicate the nature of such attachment injuries together with the EFT approach to resolving them.

THE ATTACHMENT FRAMEWORK

A clear theoretical framework on adult love is invaluable to the couple therapist. It not only helps us understand partners' wounds and difficulties and how they impact a relationship, it offers a map to effective intervention (Johnson, 2003a). Without such a framework it is often difficult to delineate the key elements of negative events and the key change events necessary to remedy them. The forgiveness literature, for example, offers little consensus as to the essential nature of specific injuries and what the critical elements are in the forgiveness process. This literature, of obvious relevance to the present topic, has not been integrated into broader theories of marriage (Coop Gordon, Baucom, & Snyder, 2000).

In attachment theory (Cassidy & Shaver, 1999), emotional bonds with a few significant others are viewed as a wired-in survival imperative. Proximity to responsive attachment figures provides us with a safe haven offering comfort and protection and a secure base, a source of confidence and security that makes exploration possible and enhances coping. Threats to these bonds activate primary fears of loss, isolation, and helplessness and amplify needs for contact comfort and soothing. In a culture that has pathologized dependency, the traumatic quality of such threats and the urgency of the protests, clinging and despair that results from them can easily be misunderstood or even considered a sign of immaturity and inadequacy.

Attachment theorists suggest further that there are only very few ways to regulate the powerful emotions that arise when the security of a bond is threatened. In the case of affairs, if the threat is manageable, if the extramarital involvement was minimal, and if the offending spouse takes responsibility and offers caring, the injured one can often reach out in the open manner typical of more secure attachment and the threat can be reduced by soothing contact and reassurance. If the threat is perceived as more serious however, or if the relationship has not offered a safe haven or secure base before the injury, then the injured spouse will either hyperactivate attachment anxieties and protests, or try to deactivate needs and fears–this results in numbing out and defensive avoidance. If injured partners are extremely fearful of both depending on and of losing their partner, these partners may swing between anxious clinging and avoidant responses. Margie, for example, would angrily protest her hurt and her spouses defensiveness and push for him to respond in a conciliatory way, but if he then responded or initiated contact, she would immediately withdraw and shut him out. As she vacillated between anxious proximity seeking and defended distancing, her spouse became more intellectual and emotionally distant. Attachment theory offers a map to the emotional realities and responses of such spouses. This allows the therapist to empathize effectively and create meaning frames that capture and order this experience.

Attachment theory also points out that models of self and other are internalized from repeated interactions with those who matter most to us. The model of the other as a dependable attachment figure, who prioritizes the spouse and the bond with the spouse, is seriously compromised by events such as affairs. This model has then to be reconstructed in couple sessions. When Margie asks, " How can I put myself in your hands again?"–part of what she is asking for is a clear narrative, an explanation of how the affair occurred and was dealt with, so that her spouse may again become known and predictable. Models of self are also threatened by these events. Margie says, "I was a fool–you made a fool of me." More importantly, she sometimes blames herself for her spouses' behavior and, in her despair, concludes that she is indeed unlovable or deficient–or he would not have turned to another. Many partners who believe that they are "strong" and should instantly end a relationship with an unfaithful spouse, have great difficulty coming to terms with their experience of vulnerability and helplessness. The EFT therapist is prepared for these responses and actively helps the client work through these fears and self-recriminations.

Attachment theory states that the essence of a secure bond is mutual emotional accessibility and responsiveness. This principle then guides the EFT therapist when he or she is helping the couple to make sense of the affair, deal with their emotions, deal with the task of forgiveness, recreate trust, and the beginnings of a renewed, more secure bond. Attachment theory and the principles of humanistic therapy on which EFT is based (Johnson, 1996; Johnson & Denton, 2002) suggest that there is no purely behavioral or predominately cognitive way of healing the hurts and injuries of events such as affairs. The strong emotions that arise must be accepted, dealt with, and then used to create specific kinds of responsive healing interactions–the kinds of interaction that are typical of the main change event in EFT–entitled a softening (Johnson, 1996), where spouses are emotionally engaged, accessible, and responsive to each other and so can comfort and soothe each other, providing an antidote to hurt and helplessness.

Before outlining the concept of attachment injuries further, I will now discuss the general EFT model, and then go on to apply this model to relationships impacted by infidelity.

THE EFT MODEL

EFT is a short-term, structured approach to the repair of distressed relationships. This approach, which is also used with families (Johnson, Maddeaux, & Blouin, 1998), has demonstrated clinical effectiveness (Johnson, Hunsley, Greenberg, & Schindler, 1999). In the most rigorous studies, 70-73% of couples were found to have recovered from distress and 90% to have significantly improved. Furthermore, there is evidence that these changes are stable and not undermined by relapse (Clothier, Manion, Gordon-Walker, & Johnson, 2002). The focus of EFT is consonant with research on the nature of marital distress by researchers such as Gottman (1994), and with the large and growing amount of research findings on adult attachment. It is also consonant with emerging themes and trends in the field of couples therapy in general. For example, it is collaborative and constructivist in nature (Johnson & Lebow, 2000; Johnson, 2003c). Furthermore, it has been successfully used in treating relationship distress that co-occurs with extreme stress due to chronic illness, depression, and posttraumatic stress disorder (Johnson & Makinen, 2003; Knowal, Johnson, & Lee, 2003). Research results suggest that level of distress at the beginning of therapy is also not a major factor in outcome. This implies that this model is appropriate for couples in crisis and severe distress.

Interventions and change processes in EFT are rooted in a clear theoretical base arising from a synthesis of the humanistic experiential, and systemic perspectives. The combination of these two perspectives allows for a focus on key emotions and on present interactional processes and patterns. The EFT perspective on close relationships is grounded in attachment theory, arguably now the most cogent theory of romantic love, and in the literature on the power of emotion to move us to action, to inform us as to what we need and want and to communicate with others. The EFT process of change is delineated into three stages, De-escalation of negative cycles, Restructuring of the emotional bond and Consolidation. These stages further delineated into nine steps. The goals of the EFT therapist are to expand constricted emotional responses that prime negative interaction patterns, restructure interactions so that partners become more accessible and responsive to each other, and foster positive cycles of comfort, caring and bonding. The therapist particularly focuses on emotion because it so potently organizes key responses to intimate others, acts as an internal compass focusing people on their primary needs and goals, and primes key meaning schemas about the nature of self and other. Negative emotional responses, such as frustration, if not attended to and restructured, undermine the repair of a couples relationship, while other "softer" emotions, such as expressions of vulnerability can be used to create new patterns of interaction. From a systemic point of view, emotion is viewed as the "leading element" in the organization of the couples interactions (Johnson, 1998).

The main change events in the second stage of EFT, withdrawer re-engagement and blamer softening, where a blaming spouse asks for his/her attachment needs for comfort and caring to be met from a position of vulnerability, result in interactions of mutual accessibility and responsiveness and more secure bonding. Process studies have outlined the steps in these change events and the main therapist interventions used (Bradley & Furrow, in press).

Infidelity may be experienced as one of many hurts in a relationship and may be addressed, as are other hurts, in the De-escalation stage by placing it in the context of the attachment history of the relationship and of specific and general negative cycles of interaction. For example, one spouse may become overwhelmed by anxiety and interrogate the "guilty" partner, who then becomes inundated with shame and hope-lessness and withdraws, leaving his partner still overwhelmed. This kind of specific cycle usually parallels the couple's general way of deal-ing with difficulties and their general negative cycle of, for example, at-tack/withdraw. In this first stage of therapy, partners are encouraged to move beyond reactive surface emotions and access their more basic at-tachment oriented emotional responses and express them to their part-ner. This occurs in relation to the infidelity as well. De-escalation is considered accomplished when both partners can see and name the cy-cles of distress and insecurity in their relationship and view these cycles as a main part of the problem. They can also then begin to address their significant hurts and fears in the relationship. If some form of infidelity is a relatively minor hurt it is then addressed as part of the usual inter-ventions in EFT. If infidelity is more significant and is experienced as a traumatizing abandonment and/or betrayal, the injured partner's an-guish and lack of trust will create impasses in Stage Two and block the change process. These injuries must then be addressed in a more fo-cused fashion and are seen as specific attachment injuries.

ATTACHMENT INJURIES

An attachment injury is defined in the EFT literature as a violation of trust resulting from a betrayal or from an abandonment at a mo-ment of intense need or vulnerability. It is a wound that violates the basic assumptions of attachment relationships. These wounds are difficult to deal with and often create an impasse in relationship re-pair. It is the attachment significance that is key—not the content of any particular incident. For a particular partner a liaison that never culminated in extra-marital sex may be as traumatic as a well estab-lished affair. For example, the client Margie, mentioned above, was traumatized by what many would consider to be a brief flirtation by her spouse. The key issue here was that this flirtation had occurred when her husband had expressed dissatisfaction with the marriage and she was taking huge risks to please him and meet his demands. The second issue was that, from Margie's perspective, he had not even considered her reaction; he had left compromising pictures of his secretary in the briefcase that she often tidied for him. This incident, as with all attachment injuries, became a pivotal moment that defined the relationship as unsafe and created an impasse in any attempt to create trust and closeness. As a result of this incident, Margie was caught in an absorbing state of anger, grief, and attachment fear, where everything led into these emotions and nothing offered a way out. She had concluded that she could never please her spouse and could never trust him again. In therapy sessions, when her husband would weep, apologize, and reach for her, her eyes would fill with tears and she would turn away. Her excessive rumination, hypervigilance, reliving or flashbacks of key scenes, alternating with numbing, and avoidance paralleled, in a less intense form, the classic symptoms of post-traumatic stress disorder.

The concept of attachment injuries was first formulated during the study of key change events in EFT, particularly Stage Two softenings. In some cases, as the EFT therapist set up a softening event, where a previously hostile spouse begins to risk being vulnerable and reach for a now available and more responsive other, the more vulnerable partner would suddenly move back to a very defended position. He or she would then refer to a particular abandonment or betrayal, announcing that because of this remembered event he or she would "never again" risk being vulnerable to the other. A series of small EFT studies are in progress to confirm the major steps in the resolution of these injuries in Stage Two of EFT, and these will be discussed below. Resolution involves not simply forgiveness between the couple but personal and interpersonal resolution to the point where reconciliation is achievable and completed softening events lead to more emotional engagement and a sense of secure bonding. The major interventions used in the resolution of these injuries are presently being studied and are hypothesized to be the same as those that facilitate softening events (Bradley & Furrow, in press), namely, heightening of key emotional responses, framing attachment needs and shaping emotional engagement with the spouse.

The key stages identified in the resolution of injuries, be they extramarital involvements or other injuries are as follows:

1. A spouse describes an incident, such as the discovery of an affair, in which he/she felt betrayed, abandoned and helpless, experiencing a violation of trust that damaged her belief in the relationship

as a secure bond. The incident is painfully alive and present rather than a calm recollection. The partner either discounts, denies, or minimizes the incident and his partner's pain and moves to a defensive stance.

2. With the therapist's help, the injured spouse stays in touch with the injury and begins to explicitly articulate its impact and its attachment significance. Newly formulated or denied emotions frequently emerge at this point. Anger often evolves into clear expressions of hurt, helplessness, fear, and shame. The connection of the injury to present negative cycles in the relationship become clear. For example, a spouse says, "I feel so wounded. I just smack him to show him he can't just wipe out my hurt. This has changed everything– I'm not sure of anything anymore. How can I let him close? I can't, even when he says he is sorry."

3. The partner supported by the therapist begins to hear and understand the significance of the wounding events and to understand them in attachment terms as a reflection of his/her importance to the injured spouse, rather than as simply a reflection of his/her personal inadequacies or "crimes." This partner then acknowledges the injured partner's pain and suffering and elaborates on how the wounding events evolved for him/her, so that his/her actions become clear and understandable to the injured partner.

4. The injured partner then tentatively moves towards a more integrated and complete articulation of the injury. With the help of the therapist, this narrative is now made clear and organized. It encapsulates the loss surrounding the injury and specific attachment fears and longings. This partner, supported by the therapist, allows the other to witness his/her vulnerability.

5. The other spouse then becomes more emotionally engaged and acknowledges responsibility for his/her part in the attachment injury/infidelity and expresses empathy, regret, and/or remorse in a congruent and emotionally engaged manner.

6. The injured spouse then risks asking for the comfort and caring from the partner that were unavailable at the time of the event, the discovery of the infidelity or the couple's previous discussions of the infidelity/injury.

7. The other spouse responds in an open caring manner that acts as an antidote to the traumatic experience of the attachment injury. The partners are then able to construct together a new narrative of the injury. This narrative is ordered and includes, for the injured spouse, a clear and acceptable sense of how the other became in-

volved with another person and how this relationship has now been resolved.

The couple then go on to build more trusting, open and emotionally healing interactions that renew and repair the bond between them and are able to move into the third consolidation phase of EFT.

If we consider the key moments in the resolution of the injury/infidelity in the client Margie's relationship, what would these key moments look like? It is first necessary to briefly describe the first few sessions of therapy. Margie and Jim describe their marriage as very distressed. Jim describes their usual way of interacting over the last 12 years, since the children were born, as "I always seem to want more connection and more sex than she does–so I guess I am always pushing for that. And she will tell you that I get real critical. But then she is an expert in shutting down and shutting me out–so I get really frustrated." Margie then quietly comments that "Nothing is ever good enough for Jim," and very gradually tells me about the "crisis" that has bought them into therapy. Twelve months before, Margie had discovered photos of Jim's secretary, posing scantily clad while sitting on his desk in his office. She found these in his briefcase while doing a clean-up of his study. She then searched his desk and found a video of an office party where this secretary was also taking off some of her clothes–ostensibly with Jim's encouragement. Jim apologized for this "indiscretion" in a short and logical fashion in the session and added that these apologies had been made regularly–to no avail–for the last year. He also added that this "flirtation," which had never evolved into a sexual affair, was "foolish" but perhaps "understandable" in light of his wife's "distance" from him. He also stated that it was time this whole issue was "fixed and over," but Margie had been "more and more distant" over the last year. I then worked with this couple to build a secure alliance, to place their present distress in the context of the above cycle and each person's attachment needs and fears. Margie was able to acknowledge that she was "reserved" and believed that adults should be self-sufficient and not talk about their emotions or "impose" on their partner. She had also come to believe that she was never going to be "special enough" for Jim and had to shut down to protect herself from his rejection. Jim was able to talk about how "desperate" he had become in the marriage for some reassurance that his wife actually needed him. He then related his "hunger" for this reassurance to his "stupid" behavior with his secretary, which he now tried to "fix" by apologizing and explaining–to no avail. Both began to see that a cycle of desperate criticism or logical "fixing of problems" from Jim and numb distancing from Margie had undermined the bond between them.

The key moments in the resolution of what Jim called the "flirtation" and what Margie called "the knife in my heart" in Stage 2 of EFT were as follows:

1. Margie is able to describe her "retreat" from Jim over the last few years and her pain at his message that she is "disappointing to him." But just before finding the photos and tape, she had become alarmed at Jim's anger at her and tried–with great trepidation–to please him by "taking risks and trying to be sexier–and more gushy." She is able to access and order her painful experience that is crystallized by his "flirtation" and to tell him–"But I can never please you–no matter how I try. And when I really went out on a limb and when I tried so hard to do everything to get you to accept me–you turned to someone else. And I died inside–I gave up. Now I just freeze around you–and your apologies are just empty words." Jim, no longer curt and logical, weeps as she speaks and tells her how much he "misses" her. Margie articulates the trauma of finding the "evidence" and her despair when Jim would try to "fix" things. She tells him, "You don't really see–care about my pain. You were willing to risk us–for a titillation." She is then able to express her grief and her need for acceptance from him.
2. Jim, who is more emotionally engaged and less "in his head" now, is able to acknowledge his demanding style and how he has made it hard for Margie to feel safe and accepted. He elaborates, in response to her questions, all the details of his "flirtation," including events that had increased his "loneliness and neediness" just before the photos and taping had occurred. He elaborates on how the flirtation evolved and how he chose not to allow it to go further. He acknowledges her pain over his actions and that in his "panic" he has been trying to force her to "get over it all." He hears and accepts her fear of being hurt again if she forgives him.
3. Margie then allows herself to express rage and also to weep openly for the anguish of "I tried so hard–I gave you what you said you wanted–and right then–you risked us–you turned to her to feel good–like I didn't matter–I am broken–devastated." And Jim is able to stay engaged and hear her. She tells him that letting him in has to be slow–that he cannot demand that she shape up to his expectations in this.

4. Jim is more and more able to stay emotionally engaged with Margie rather than become impatient, rationalize, and imply that her responses are unreasonable. He is able to express his remorse and regret at the hurt he caused her and acknowledge her right to her self-protective responses. He is able to tell Margie that he wants now to help her feel safe and accepted and give her the reassurance she needs.
5. Margie, step by step, is able to move from, " I don't know what I need now" to asserting that she needs Jim's "acceptance" and to "know I am precious to him–even if I am not as out there as he is–or as other women can be."
6. Jim is able to comfort and reassure his wife and talk of how it has been easier to "pressure" her than to acknowledge his own loneliness and that she is like "life itself" to him.

Once the process above has been completed, the couple move into Consolidation and are able to create a narrative of how they repaired their bond and how Margie was able to forgive Jim his "flirtation" and risk with him again. They were also able to make concrete plans to enhance their intimacy and help each other with their "needs and fears."

CONCLUSION

The EFT therapist believes that infidelity and other relational crises are best seen in the context adult attachment. Attachment is an integrative theory. It is a theory of affect regulation; it is a systemic theory that looks at cyclical patterns of responses but it also encompasses basic universal intrapsychic needs and fears; it is a theory of trauma–the trauma of loss and isolation. A focus on key emotions and their attachment significance allows the therapist to shape the process of forgiveness and the creation, and perhaps for the first time, of a secure attachment bond.

REFERENCES

Bowlby, J. (1969). *Attachment and loss: Vol. 1. Attachment.* New York: Basic
Bowlby, J. (1988). *A secure base.* New York: Basic.
Bradley, B., & Furrow, J. (in press) Toward a mini-theory of EFT therapist behaviors facilitating a softening event. *Journal of Marital & Family Therapy.*
Cassidy, J., & Shaver, P. (Eds.). (1999) *Handbook of attachment: Theory, research, and clinical implications.* New York: Guilford Press.

Clothier, P., Manion, I., Gordon Walker, J., & Johnson, S. M. (2002) Emotionally focused interventions for couples with chronically ill children, *Journal of Marital & Family Therapy*, 28, 391-399 .

Coop Gordon, K., Baucom, D. S., & Snyder, D. K. (2000) The use of forgiveness in marital therapy. In M. McCullough, K., Pargament, K. I., & C. E. Thoresen (Eds.), *Forgiveness: Theory, Research, & Practice*, pp. 203-227. New York: Guilford Press.

Gottman, J. (1994) *What predicts divorce?* Hillsdale, NJ: Erlbaum.

Greenberg, L. S., & Johnson, S. M. (1988) *Emotionally focused therapy for couples*. New York: Guilford Press.

Johnson, S. M. (1996). *The practice of emotionally focused marital therapy: Creating connection.* New York: Brunner/Mazel (now Brunner/Routledge).

Johnson, S. M. (1998). Listening to the music: Emotion as a natural part of systems theory. *Journal of Systemic Therapies*, 17, 1-18.

Johnson, S. M. (2002). *Emotional couples therapy for trauma survivors: Strengthening attachment bonds.* New York: Guilford Press.

Johnson, S. M. (2003 a). Introduction to attachment: A therapist's guide to primary relationships and their renewal. In S. M. Johnson & V. Whiffen (Eds.), *Attachment processes in couple & family therapy*, pp. 3-17. New York: Guilford Press.

Johnson, S. M. (2003 b). Attachment theory: A guide for couple therapy. In S. M. Johnson & V. Whiffen (Eds.), *Attachment processes in couple & family therapy*, pp. 103- 123. New York: Guilford Press.

Johnson, S. M. (2003 c). The revolution in couples therapy: A practitioner-scientist perspective. *Journal of Marital & Family Therapy,* 29, 365-384.

Johnson, S. M., & Denton, W. (2002). Emotionally focused couples therapy: Creating secure connections. In A. Gurman & N. Jacobson (Eds.), *Clinical Handbook of Couple Therapy*, pp. 221-250. New York: Guilford Press.

Johnson, S., Hunsley, J., Greenberg, L. S., & Schlindler, D. (1999). The effects of emotionally focused marital therapy: A meta-analysis. *Clinical Psychology: Science and Practice,* 6, 67-79.

Johnson, S. M., & Lebow, J. (2000). The coming of age of couple therapy: A decade review. *Journal of Marital & Family Therapy,* 26, 23-38.

Johnson, S.M., Maddeaux, C., & Blouin, J. (1998). Emotionally focused family therapy for bulimia: Changing attachment patterns. *Psychotherapy,* 35, 238-247.

Johnson, S. M., Makinen, J. A., & Millikin, J. W. (2001). Attachment injuries in couple relationships: A new perspective on impasses in couples therapy. *Journal of Marital & Family Therapy,* 27, 145-155.

Johnson, S. M., & Makinen, J. (2003). Posttraumatic Stress. In D. K. Snyder & M. A. Whisman (Eds.), *Treating difficult couples,* pp. 308-329. New York: Guilford Press.

Knowal, J., Johnson, S. M., & Lee, A. (2003). Chronic illness in couples: A case for Emotionally Focused Therapy. *Journal of Marital & Family Therapy,* 29, 299-310.

Whisman, M.A., Dixon, A. E., & Johnson, B. (1997). Therapists perspectives of couple problems and treatment issues in couple therapy. *Journal of Family Psychology,* 11, 361-366.

Undercurrents

David Moultrup

SUMMARY. In a story-telling mode, with a personal and intimate fla-
vor, this article takes a look at one approach to the treatment of an extramarital affair. With roots in Bowen theory, and an attention to the
underlying dynamics of the emotional system, the treatment is further
enriched by an improvisational approach which acknowledges the self
of therapist. *[Article copies available for a fee from The Haworth Document
Delivery Service: 1-800-HAWORTH. E-mail address: <docdelivery@
haworthpress.com> Website: <http://www.HaworthPress.com> © 2005 by The
Haworth Press, Inc. All rights reserved.]*

KEYWORDS. Infidelity, Bowen theory, self of therapist, long-term
treatment

"We *really* need help. Can we come in to see you as soon as possible?" The voice on the phone has a familiar ring of sadness and despera-
tion. I have a strong sense I know what's coming. My hunch is quickly
confirmed when she continues.

"My husband is involved with another woman. We haven't slept in
days, we're up talking all night. We obviously need someone to help us
through this."

Address correspondence to: David Moultrup, MSW, LICSW, 5 Watson Road, Belmont,
MA 02478 (E-mail: dmoultrup@verizon.net).

[Haworth co-indexing entry note]: "Undercurrents." Moultrup, David. Co-published simultaneously in
Journal of Couple & Relationship Therapy (The Haworth Press) Vol. 4, No. 2/3, 2005, pp. 31-40; and: *Handbook of the Clinical Treatment of Infidelity* (ed: Fred P. Piercy, Katherine M. Hertlein, and Joseph L.
Wetchler) The Haworth Press, Inc., 2005, pp. 31-40. Single or multiple copies of this article are available for a
fee from The Haworth Document Delivery Service [1-800-HAWORTH, 9:00 a.m. - 5:00 p.m. (EST). E-mail
address: docdelivery@haworthpress.com].

Available online at http://www.haworthpress.com/web/JCRT
© 2005 by The Haworth Press, Inc. All rights reserved.
doi:10.1300/J398v04n02_04

The glut of songs, movies, books, and poetry that focus on affairs are a testament to the intense feelings they trigger. Whether it's the feelings of the main characters in the drama, or of family members, friends, neighbors, co-workers, uninvolved onlookers, and occasionally even the therapist, there is no end to the many facets that invite probing.

"As I said over the phone, Greg has become involved with another woman. I don't want the marriage to end. We don't know what to do." The first session picks up where the phone call stopped. Lisa opens the session with a clear signal about her willingness to work on the marriage.

"I've tried to tell Lisa that I didn't intend for this to happen, but it just did. At this point I don't know whether we can make the marriage work or not." Greg's entry into the discussion lays out two of the critical elements, that he hadn't been looking for another involvement, and that now that it is here, he is highly skeptical about the viability of the marriage.

My role in this drama is something that I have explored for years, and written about in-depth (Moultrup, 1990). I have considered it a profound responsibility and honor to find some way to use myself as a positive voice as the crisis of an affair plays out in the life of a couple. I am continually humbled by the notion that there is something in the process of exploration that can have an impact on the course of people's lives.

Having struggled with so many people in the midst of this crisis for many decades, I still never know how any given couple will make its way through the turbulence, or in what way I will make a difference. I am convinced there is no one simple formula for treatment, no one simple classification scheme for affairs, and no one set of labels that adequately describes the characters in the drama. Constructs of this nature are designed to manage the anxiety of those discussing the situation and fulfill media needs for catchy labels.

I find myself in awe of the depth and breadth of fundamental life forces which are at play in the dynamics of an affair. These crises, which are among the most common of crises in a marriage, are not about secretive trysts in romantic settings, and not about the poorly conceived notion of sexual addiction. They're not even really about the gut-wrenching feelings of betrayal when the liaison comes to light, or the fear of recommitment. Certainly, many of these experiences command attention, and helpful therapy will handle those moments. Focusing only on those elements, however, will do a disservice to the couple, and a disservice to the complexity of the core dynamics which are inevitably at work.

The basics of life are lurking beneath the attention-getting lies and tears. Showing the way to the exploration of these undercurrents, these unseen foundations, will become one of the primary goals of the therapy. That work will aim at the potential of giving clients the vision to make informed and mature decisions about the course of their own lives. It will also look toward a process of healing the feelings which will saturate the crisis, and healing older feelings, indeed a lifetime's worth, which likely fed into the early root system of the affair.

I usually find it helpful to have both individual and conjoint sessions with a couple. Individual sessions give me an opportunity to know different dimensions of each person and give them an opportunity to explore parts of themselves they don't understand. Ultimately these insights make it back to the conjoint sessions, where the individual can engage with their partner about them.

I asked Greg about his own feelings a bit later in the first session. "Have you considered simply leaving the marriage? It seems like you're not at all sure it is working for you." Greg's response is strong, "At this point I don't know what to do. I know I've found something with Diane that I've never had with Lisa. But leaving Lisa and the kids is a very tough decision. I'm not ready to do that."

This was a signal to me there was still a strong emotional bond between Greg and Lisa. This was not the time to separate. It was, instead, a time to help both of them become more clear about the meaning of the crisis on both an individual and systemic level, and the implications for their future either together or separate.

In a later individual session I asked Greg to explain what he had found with Diane. His response was tentative, but showed thought. "I've recently come to understand that I didn't like the me that existed in my relationship with Lisa. I feel like a different person when I'm with Diane." Sometimes I choose to let certain topics pass by in any given session, but this one I immediately took up. This observation opened the door to perhaps the most central of all of the foundation themes, the issue of self.

This, of course, is a multifaceted notion which isn't simply outlined in one sitting. Typical of all of the important themes in therapy, Greg and I would return to this one regularly, with him gaining more clarity with each foray into the territory. Invariably, there are multigenerational roots which need to be understood to truly facilitate change. My challenge to him was to gain clarity about what parts of himself seemed to be most evident with each different woman.

Interventions during this process are spontaneous. The actual doing of therapy for me is a creative exchange, disciplined by theory and catalyzed by the ability to make use of what the patient brings, what I bring, and the moment of the encounter. It draws upon the same skills I have developed as an improvising musician. In that way, it is an artistic pursuit more than a technical series of steps to follow.

Meanwhile, Lisa was in acute distress. She, too, displayed a thoughtfulness and even a willingness to take on some responsibility. "I truly believe that Greg would not have gotten involved in this relationship if everything was OK between us." Lisa's observation in a joint session was a fertile clue that she was able to understand some kind of systemic component to the affair. I made a mental note that I would need to monitor the balance between her willingness to see the impact of the marriage, and understanding that there is part of this crisis that is about unresolved tensions in Greg that have nothing to do with her.

But her observation did trigger an exploration of the evolution of their relationship. Greg and Lisa agreed that theirs was a difficult history. They became involved in the wake of troubled previous relationships, and believed that theirs was a rebound for both of them. There was frequent conflict from the start, much of it centering around whether they should continue, not continue, get married, and have children. They did get married and have children, but Greg's image of himself through the years was one of chronic unhappiness. Lisa agreed.

This troubled history is somewhat of an eyebrow raising theme in the therapy. This style is in sharp contrast to a history in which both partners agree that indeed the relationship was a good one when it first started, but things went downhill. This contrasting image, which emerges with careful history-taking, reveals an initial period of time that worked well. This pattern declines, with pressures contributing to escalating tension in the marriage. These often include the death of a parent or other significant family member, job loss, or other major life change.

While the history of the marriage is significant to the crisis at hand, their respective histories with their families of origin are critical as well. Having looked over their relationship, Greg and Lisa were easily drawn into an examination of their earlier background. There were significant themes on both sides.

Lisa acknowledged from the start that she now understood that one of the problems that had existed between her and Greg was her strong feelings of obligation to her family. She often found herself caring for her parents, frequently to the detriment of time with her husband and children. She made a very strong point that she knew she needed to reorganize her priorities in this way, and began a very conscious program to re-balance that part of her life. The challenge would be to retain a good relationship with her parents, all the while giving a higher priority to her current family. Although Lisa's recognition of the need for change was significant, it was clear that a careful exploration of the issue of differentiation would be useful as the therapy progressed.

Greg's history was equally significant, but in a different way. As Greg began relaying his history, he began with his father. "I don't have a lot do to with my dad at this point. He lives far away, and things have never been the same since he left." His parents had divorced when he was ten years old. His father left the family for another woman. It was very clear that Greg had intense feelings about his dad and their history together. These feelings would be too complex to untangle in one conversation. It would take considerable work.

One of the ways that I think of Greg in relation to his father is to think of the situation as a triangle between Greg, his dad, and Diane, the other woman. A key component of Bowen theory (Bowen, 1978), the notion of triangles offers yet another one of the key undercurrents in the dynamics of affairs. Strange as it may seem, the obvious triangle of Greg, Lisa, and Diane is not the most significant triangle to understand.

Yes, there is a triangle between Greg, Lisa, and Diane. And the fact that this triangle exists is the precipitating crisis for entering therapy. Likewise, it is this triangle which is the usual focus for much of the artistic and media focus. But emotional triangles exist between any three people in a family system. Some of them end up having more emotional impact than others.

Greg's complex feelings about his father act almost like an energy system. His antagonism towards him, coupled with the natural tendencies to emulate a parent, create an internal struggle for Greg. In part, his attraction to Diane seemed to be an unconscious desire on his part to re-capitulate his father's history. In the face of a barrage of negative images Greg lives with concerning his father, there is an undercurrent of him being utterly compelled to follow in his footsteps.

In that way, neither Lisa nor Diane are central to this part of the drama, despite the natural inclination for him to make a list of the advantages and disadvantages of the two relationships. In this case, as with most, it is clear that the women are different from each other. It is also true that Greg feels different with each, and that he believes a different part of himself is accessible in the different relationships.

But in a way which pre-dates his relationship with either woman, and seems to preempt those dynamics, there are the dynamics with his father. His unmet needs for connection, mentoring, support, and love from his father seem to be playing out in part by repeating his father's life course, and in that way becoming closer, or more like, his father.

Is Greg compelled to have his life script defined by following in his father's footsteps? This is the work of the therapy. In a bigger way, this triangle is but one of many interlocking triangles throughout the emotional system which have a bearing on the affair. The exploration of them will be a subtle but powerful component of the therapy.

I am sure that it is clear to the reader at this point that this story has many different facets, none of which have been remotely clarified. This is a very intentional mirroring of the process of the therapy. The focus of the therapy will flow between the present, the history of the couple, and the multigenerational themes, depending on the accessibility of the moment.

Lisa asked a question that arises frequently. "How long does it take to resolve this kind of crisis?" It came during a joint session in the context of a discussion about stress. She wished, she said, that she could wake up and have this crisis be over. My answer to her, with a tone of somber compassion and support, reveals the part of this no one ever likes to hear, "Longer than you want it to." Human nature is such that these ordeals take a long time to truly work out. People need both calendar time and therapy time to come to resolution.

This can often be a problem as it relates to the turn-of-the-millennium health-care model. People who become involved in affairs are generally not flagrantly psychotic, suicidal, or in the throes of a biologically based disorder. Insurance companies often decide that therapy is therefore "not medically indicated." In fact, therapy is vital to assist them through the crisis. But the social context of third-party payment for those services has been severely compromised. Couples might choose to pass on therapy rather than pay their own way. Lisa and Greg saw that it had something to offer, and they return week after week as we go deeper into the roots of the affair.

One of the challenging and creative parts of the therapy is weaving together the exploration of the undercurrents with the management of the daily drama. Lisa brought up one of the most common sub-plots in an individual session. "I know that Greg is continuing to see Diane. I don't know how I should handle it." While the multigenerational themes will be core to eventual resolution, there is the very real need to address the mounting tension created between Greg and Lisa about his involvement with Diane.

My answer to this question, again, is more difficult and ambiguous than anyone would prefer. "Ultimately, if we are going to do any real work on the marriage, Greg obviously has to totally end things with Diane. But unfortunately it does neither you nor I any good to try to demand it. It puts us in the role of trying to police his behavior, which is impossible." It's useful that Lisa brought up this problem in an individual session. It gives me an opportunity to join with her concerning the dilemma.

"So what can we do with this, then?" Lisa's tone tells me that she is receptive to the idea, sees the sense of it, but is still left with uncertainty.

"For a while, you're going to have to be the one letting us know how much you can take. We're all going to know that Greg is still involved with Diane. I'm sure there's a lot of work we can do while that continues. But if you get to a point where you are too frustrated, you need to let me know." My answer to Lisa is designed to address both the feelings that I know she'll be having, yet engage her thinking in such a way as to get objectivity, and an increased ability to tolerate working in an ambiguous context.

More often than not, couples that find their way into my office are at a point in the emotional hurricane of an affair that it would do no good to demand an end to the affair, demand an end to the marriage, or demand an end to therapy. Neither relationship is going to end on demand. Ending the therapy implies that there is no therapeutic benefit to offer at this stage of the crisis. I am clear that my approach to therapy has much to offer at this stage.

We continue to explore the various areas already mentioned. Returning to the balance in the marriage prior to the affair helps to gain considerable clarity about the unhealthy dynamics which fed into the problems. One theme which emerged as truly significant was that of power. In both joint sessions and individual sessions, it became clear that Greg felt less powerful than Lisa. Although both of them had successful careers, Greg's work brought a lower financial payoff than Lisa's did. Also, Lisa had a cushion of a family inheritance which further contributed to her financial stability.

Lisa, on her part, had not felt like she was using the money as a power base in the marriage. Quite to the contrary. She simply felt like she had used the resources as a way to maintain the financial solvency of the family. Greg, on the other hand, though he hadn't really known it consciously, had clearly felt a chronic sense of inadequacy and discomfort, experiencing a sense of disempowerment with his perception of the imbalance.

As the issue of power got developed over time, it became clear to me that both Greg and Lisa felt weak in the relationship. Lisa felt frustrated at her inability to engage Greg in a more comprehensive involvement in the family. She often ended up making decisions without Greg because she was unable to get his input on the decision. Greg, on the other hand, saw Lisa as the one in control of most of family life.

Conversely, it became equally clear that his relationship with Diane was the reverse of this situation. With Diane, he was clearly the dominant person and the one who provided the most resources to the relationship. The theme of Greg's definition of self clearly was core to this powerful dynamic undercurrent.

Despite Greg's disaffection from Lisa, and despite his obvious emotional entanglement with Diane, he was not able to be decisive about discontinuing the marriage. He sent signals to Lisa in sessions and out of sessions that he still cared for her, and didn't want to destroy the family. These usually came across as recollecting his love of Lisa from years gone by.

Even more complex was his position regarding the children, in which there was a clear and ongoing sense of contradiction and paradox. On the one hand, he constantly expressed agony that he didn't want to do to his children what his dad had done to him. On the other hand, there was a sense of inevitability and pressure to recapitulate his father's choice which was ever present.

A profound difference began to emerge between them. While Lisa saw the history and acknowledged the trouble, she was steadfast in her belief that the new knowledge of the multigenerational themes could enable them to create a new and healthier relationship. In the background of her position was her family's history of intact relationships and very few divorces.

Greg, on the other hand, was unable to re-engage emotionally with Lisa. He had a sense of the possibility of his need to re-trace his father's footsteps. But his attachment to Diane, and his perception of his uncomfortable balance with Lisa, drew him further out of the marriage. He chose to move out of the house after a period of time. The initial choice was prompted by a desire to decrease the level of conflict between them. It was an open question at that point as to whether the marriage could be rehabilitated.

After leaving, Greg remained in contact with Lisa and the children, and also remained emotionally closed off from Lisa. The continued couples' work enabled Lisa to see the nature of Greg's disengagement from her as a function not only of their time together, but of Greg's early history as well. Eventually Lisa made the choice to initiate the divorce process, despite her fundamental desire to maintain the marriage. She could see that Greg simply was unable to return to her emotionally.

The fact that it was Lisa who ultimately made the move towards divorce was a telling manifestation of the core power dynamic which had been revealed throughout the marriage. Lisa clearly wanted Greg back. In the absence of decisive steps on his part, Lisa made the choice, steeled against the inevitable difficulties it would precipitate. While it was possible for Greg to proclaim that here, again, it was Lisa who was "in charge," it was clear that his lack of assertion was central to the outcome.

The work with Greg and Lisa extended over more than two years. This period of time is typical for this type of crisis. Over that time, both of them had bouts of depression, and were put on anti-depressant medication. Each of them clearly found the therapy very helpful, and each highly valued the therapeutic relationship with me. Both expressed much gratitude for the structure of integrating conjoint sessions with individual sessions. The process helped them both untangle the meaning of the chaos in their lives over the period of the treatment. It helped create a structure for the process of separation which took place.

While the marriage did not survive, it seems too simplistic to characterize the affair as Greg's vehicle to escape a bad marriage. The powerful multigenerational themes suggest a more fundamental, bedrock process of definition of self which was at the base of the crisis. Until the very end, Lisa was insistent on the potential to rebuild the relationship. Until the very end, Greg was unable to own a sense of empowerment and reengage emotionally with Lisa.

One of the notions in the Bowen model is that people tend to choose mates of equal levels of differentiation. It would be possible to sketch out the balance between Greg and Lisa to fit this model. But their experience, and many like it, pose a difficult question about the premise. Did Lisa show a greater ability to grow and learn, perhaps a greater level of differentiation? What does this mean about her basic sense of self? The question could be explored relative to the entire history between Lisa and Greg.

And there are other questions which inevitably will emerge as everyone moves into a new stage of life. Will Greg be able to create a more healthy relationship with Diane than he did with Lisa? What kind of relationship will he maintain with his children? What kind of benefits will he ultimately gain from the divorce?

The opportunity to wrestle with these questions and others are at the heart of the professional and personal satisfaction which has kept me fulfilled for so many decades of engaging with couples in the midst of a crisis. I haven't taken my job to be one of saving marriages, though more often than not that has been the outcome. For me, the role of the therapist is one of facilitating human growth. It comes from a combination of offering potential routes through difficult terrain, offering different perspectives and ways of understanding, and helping to gain clarity about the many undercurrents which are contributing to life.

REFERENCES

Bowen, M. (1978). *Family therapy in clinical practice.* NY: Jason Aronson
Moultrup, D. J. (1990). *Husbands, wives, and lovers: The emotional system of the extra-marital affair.* NY: Guilford

Healing the Wounds of Infidelity Through the Healing Power of Apology and Forgiveness

Brian Case

SUMMARY. This article focuses on a treatment model for couples dealing with the consequences of an extra-relational affair by one of the partners. The model is based around a multi-dimensional process of apology and forgiveness, in which each spouse works toward the restoration or relational trust through specific tasks. Examples from the author's private practice are used to help clarify key concepts and aid in application across various situations. *[Article copies available for a fee from The Haworth Document Delivery Service: 1-800-HAWORTH. E-mail address: <docdelivery@haworthpress.com> Website: <http://www.HaworthPress.com> © 2005 by The Haworth Press, Inc. All rights reserved.]*

KEYWORDS. Infidelity, restoration of trust, apology, forgiveness, treatment model

Brian Case, PhD, is affiliated with Psychological Counseling Services, Ltd., Scottsdale, AZ 85251.

[Haworth co-indexing entry note]: "Healing the Wounds of Infidelity Through the Healing Power of Apology and Forgiveness." Case, Brian. Co-published simultaneously in *Journal of Couple & Relationship Therapy* (The Haworth Press) Vol. 4, No. 2/3, 2005, pp. 41-54; and: *Handbook of the Clinical Treatment of Infidelity* (ed: Fred P. Piercy, Katherine M. Hertlein, and Joseph L. Wetchler) The Haworth Press, Inc., 2005, pp. 41-54. Single or multiple copies of this article are available for a fee from The Haworth Document Delivery Service [1-800-HAWORTH, 9:00 a.m. - 5:00 p.m. (EST). E-mail address: docdelivery@ haworthpress.com].

Available online at http://www.haworthpress.com/web/JCRT
© 2005 by The Haworth Press, Inc. All rights reserved.
doi:10.1300/J398v04n02_05

I have always told myself, my friends, and my husband Tom that if he ever cheated on me–that would be it, no questions asked. And yet although I'm not sure why, I'm not quite ready to walk away.

This statement, in so many words, has been repeated by numerous clients over the past 7 years that I have been specializing in working with couples facing the aftermath of one partner's extra-relational affair, or ERA. Indeed, most of my clients report that they assumed they would be meeting with a divorce attorney, not a marital therapist, following the discovery of an affair. When a couple begins therapy following one partner's infidelity, it can be difficult for the marriage and family therapist to know where to begin. Nevertheless, because of the prevalence of this presenting problem, a treatment format through which the post-affair couple can find healing, and possibly a renewed sense of commitment and trust, is of great value.

The following article presents one means of doing so, specifically through a comprehensive, interactive process of reconciliation focused on apology and forgiveness. The steps or "tasks" of the processes of forgiveness and apology as outlined here have been developed over the past 10 years through a combination of a detailed review of literature on forgiveness done for my doctoral dissertation, and clinical experience as a full-time therapist in private practice. Key literature regarding the conceptualization of forgiveness as a process includes Donnelly (1966), Rosenak and Harnden (1992), Smedes (1983), Hargrave (1995), Enright (1989), and Simon and Simon (1990).

WHY APOLOGY AND FORGIVENESS?

When a couple seeks counseling after an affair, they face a wide variety of intense emotions and difficult decisions. One of the most common questions is whether or not trust can ever be restored, and if so, how? For the betrayed partner, it may seem an impossible journey to move from anger to forgiveness, from mistrust to reconciliation, and from broken heart to healing. One client expressed this sense of being overwhelmed in saying "one minute I feel incredible sadness and rejection and the next I feel like ripping his head off. . . . I can't imagine this pain ever ending!" Furthermore, I frequently hear clients say "I can't believe I didn't see this. . . how did I let this happen?" They feel vulnerable, defective, and unable to trust themselves as well as their partners. In her book, *After the Affair*, Spring (1997) describes how betrayed partners suddenly feel as if they've lost, among many things, their identity, sense of "specialness," self-respect, and sense of purpose. For the involved partner the journey can also seem impossible. He or she is likely dealing not only with the damage to his/her primary relationship, but is also going through a grieving process as the affair has come, or is coming, to an end. Therefore, for each partner there is a need for a specific plan of action that allows for the healing of existing wounds, the prevention of future wounds, and the restoration of trust and vitality to the relationship.

FORGIVENESS DEFINED

Work in the areas of apology and forgiveness allows couples to accomplish these three goals. Forgiveness is defined here as a complex, multidimensional, multi-modal process consisting of at least four distinguishable levels or degrees, including:

1. Ceasing to Seek/Demand Justice or Revenge
2. Ceasing to Feel Anger/Resentment
3. Wishing the Other Person Well
4. Restoring Relational Trust

Initially then, forgiveness is about choosing to not actively hurt the other person back, demand or suggest that somebody else hurt him/her, or to hope or perhaps even pray that the person suffers somehow. The ancient Chinese proverb that "he who chooses revenge as an option has need of digging two graves" clarifies one benefit of this level of forgiveness. The second level involves working through the hurt, pain, anger and resentment to the point where these emotions have dissipated significantly. The benefits of the 3rd level of forgiveness are at times difficult to see, and yet are critical nonetheless. Indeed, as Hope (1987) points out, when anger and perhaps hatred are replaced with compassion or well-wishing for the other person, the "giver" of this gift is usually the one most benefited.

These first 3 levels can be experienced regardless of how apologetic the offending person is. However, when significant betrayal has occurred such as in the case of an ERA, the 4th level of forgiveness is usually dependent on the degree to which the partner engages in some process of apology. It is forgiveness work geared toward this last level that is the focus of the remainder of this article. In the following sections, I will present comprehensive processes of forgiveness and apology that may be used with the post-affair couple.

SETTING THE STAGE

When a couple has stated that they want to somehow recover from the affair and stay together, I will introduce the topics of apology and forgiveness by exploring their thoughts and feelings on the topic, and then sharing with them ways in which such work might be helpful. If agreeable to both, I will then provide information on the processes of apology and forgiveness as outlined in Table 1, and ask each to start an on-going letter to his/her partner based on the tasks identified in the handout. The betrayed spouse will be using the Process of Forgiveness as an outline, while the involved spouse will use the Process of Apology.

I explain that the idea is to work on the letters over the course of therapy, as the work of healing unfolds. I clarify that by the time they actually share the letters with one another, several weeks to months, and a lot of "blood, sweat, and tears" will have come and gone. In this sense the letters are not the means to healing and reconciliation, but a final concrete representation of the journey taken, the work done, and the healing experienced.

Recognizing/Acknowledging the Injustice(s)

For many clients, the work of recognizing and acknowledging how they have been hurt through their partner's affair is done long before

TABLE 1. The Process of Forgiveness

1. Recognizing/acknowledging the injustice(s).
2. Choosing forgiveness as an option.
3. Getting in touch with feelings of hurt/anger.
4. Expressing the feelings in non-hurtful ways.
5. Gaining insights which allow for self-protection.
6. Gaining insights which allow you to focus on the behavior, not the person.
7. Recognizing your own role in the "bigger picture" of hurtful behaviors in the relationship.
8. Using new information to change how you view and treat the hurtful person.
9. The overt act of forgiveness and restoration of love and trust.

therapy begins. However, there are many situations in which the betrayed partner does not yet know everything about the affair, or has not yet felt the full impact of what is already known. Therefore, the focus of this task is to make sure all of the "wounds" have been identified so complete healing can ultimately occur. Too often, perhaps motivated by a desire to minimize pain, parts of the ERA which constitute significant hurts within the overall betrayal of the affair go unaddressed. For instance, the seemingly steady progress of one couple was delayed after the husband disclosed to his wife for the first time that his sexual involvement with the other woman had resulted in a pregnancy which was terminated through abortion. For her, this was the more difficult act of betrayal to overcome.

Therapists can help each partner identify these different levels of betrayal asking questions regarding how the affair came to the knowledge of the betrayed partner, whether or not the relationship was on-going or short term, whether or not exchanges of "I love you" or plans to "run off together" were made, whether or not money was spent on the other person, whether or not intimate details of their relationship were shared with the other person, or whether or not sexual protection was used. The degree of harmful impact on the betrayed partner is also influenced by factors such as where and how did the betrayal take place? For one betrayed spouse, the most damaging blow was the fact that her husband left the hospital after their second child was born to sleep with his girlfriend. For another, it was the fact that his wife had been sexual with her lover in their lakeside cabin, a place both had seen as their "sanctuary."

Choosing Forgiveness as an Option

Through the work of uncovering layers of betrayal, many betrayed partners begin to lose their desire for reconciliation. For this reason, the work of the next task, choosing forgiveness as an option, is likely to be revisited throughout the entire process. Helping the betrayed partner understand the levels of forgiveness as outlined above can be helpful. As therapists, we can point out that choosing forgiveness initially is not necessarily a commitment to stay in the relationship no matter what, but is instead a decision to give healing a chance. Clearly, it is not only the betrayed partner who has to decide whether or not to try and reconcile. Many of the couples I work with are facing the extremely difficult task of trying to rebuild trust when one of the two still has strong feelings for another person. When present, this challenge needs to be identified and discussed openly in either individual or couples sessions.

Getting in Touch with Feelings of Hurt/Anger

In order to recover from an affair, each partner has to be willing to face the painful emotional work inherent to the journey. Indeed, the task of getting in touch with emotions is the easiest part of forgiveness work for many individuals. They do not need to be encouraged to "get in touch with their anger" but instead feel as if they are about to explode with rage (if they haven't already done so!). However, many clients will present in a state of emotional disconnect due to the shock of the affair. Furthermore, there are a surprising number of people who remain emotionally disconnected due to long-standing coping mechanisms in which intense, "negative" emotions are avoided at all costs, often outside of their conscious awareness. The emotion of anger in particular is often repressed by the betrayed spouse due to fears of rejection and abandonment. This is often accompanied by engaging in "outreach" instead of "outrage," a pattern I frequently see in which intense feelings of love, appreciation and sexual desire are expressed despite the recent crisis.

Therefore, in-session interventions are often necessary to help clients begin the emotional work of forgiveness. These can include pointing out patterns of emotional repression when present, providing education about and "normalization" of intense emotions, and encouraging the exploration of emotions through journal writing, bibliotherapy, or talking with friends or family members. Experiential therapy techniques can also be helpful in both the identification and healthy expression of feelings surrounding the affair.

Expressing the Feelings in Non-Hurtful Ways

While a great deal of emotional expression may have already taken place before therapy began, it is likely that not all qualified as "non-hurtful." For instance, in one of our weekly "Anger and Forgiveness" group sessions, a 52-year-old woman told of how she emptied her husband's side of the closet by throwing his expensive clothing out the window of the two-story home, onto the wet, winter grass which had recently been fertilized with cow manure. Other group members cheered her on, and I myself had to fight off a smile at the thought of this usually quiet and very "appropriate" woman exacting her revenge. However, her behavior was aggressive and shaming, and in the long run did not contribute to healing for her or for the relationship. (It in fact later became a part of her apology work within the relationship!)

Therefore, it is critical as therapists to help the betrayed partner express anger and other intense emotions to his/her partner assertively, rather than through verbal or physical aggression. Techniques for expressing feelings while alone should also be identified. For one client writing raw, unedited letters on the computer and then deleting them afterwards was very cathartic. For another, smashing inexpensive dishes (purchased at a garage sale for that very purpose) into a large metal trash can in their backyard helped her work through anger triggered by mental flashbacks of walking in on her husband and his girlfriend.

Gaining Insights Which Allow for Self-Protection

While forgiveness work involves working through considerable pain, it is not about creating it. As Hargrave (1988), emphasizes, there is room for appropriate self-protection within the forgiveness process. Many of my clients wonder out loud, "how could I have let this happen?" or express that they "feel like such a fool!" They may have ignored intuitions about something being wrong, concluding that they "must be crazy." The loss of trust in self as well as in the partner often leaves the betrayed partner in a state of confusion and overprotection.

Indeed, many people are hesitant to seek forgiveness as an option for fear that to do so will result in a greater likelihood of getting hurt again. Therefore, the main goal within this task is for the betrayed partner to learn the specific ways in which his/her partner was able to "pull it off." As therapists, we can also encourage and support the betrayed partner to identify ways in which he/she may have enabled the affair unknowingly. These insights can then inform decisions about what boundaries need to be in place in the name of assertive self-protection. These boundaries, unlike "emotional walls," allow for both connection *and* protection.

Gaining Insights Which Allow You to Focus on the Behavior, Not the Person

For betrayed partners, there is a strong tendency to see themselves and/or their partners as "damaged goods." "Only a monster could do something so hurtful," or "I'm obviously not good enough for him/her" are common sentiments. Therefore, the task here is to look at the betrayal within the context it occurred. Doing so helps the betrayed partner recognize that while the involved partner's infidelity was personally damaging, it does not have to be "taken personal." I knew one client had discovered this for herself when after weeks of feeling "less-than" as a woman, she emphatically claimed, "It wasn't about me, it was about his unhealthy need for validation by other women. . . I think he could have been married to a supermodel and still ended up sleeping around."

It is also important to help the betrayed partner recognize how the involved partner's family background, learned coping mechanisms, insecurities, cognitive distortions, etc., have factored in to him/her engaging in such hurtful behaviors. It can help to asks questions such as "which of his/her life experiences, if different somehow, might have resulted in him/her being less likely to make such hurtful choices?" Through such a question, and his subsequent openness to learning more about his wife's sexual abuse background and personal struggles with shame, one client was able to release his desire to, as he put it, "rub her face in it daily."

Recognizing Your Own Role in the "Bigger Picture" of Hurtful Behaviors in the Relationship

A focus on the relational context in which the affair occurred can often be helpful in the reconciliation process. The work of this task is for the betrayed partner to make an honest acknowledgement of his/her own weaknesses and need for forgiveness. One betrayed wife experienced a change in heart as she more fully recognized how, although she could never see herself cheating, she had created considerable damage over the course of the relationship through abusive name-calling, being active in her eating disorder, and being shut-down sexually. These behaviors were coupled with her unwillingness to go to counseling, despite his frequent requests.

Using New Information to Change How You View and Treat the Hurtful Person

The work of seeing the affair within context helps lay the groundwork for a shift into the third level of forgiveness, "wishing the other person well." While this shift into compassion may occur naturally throughout the forgiveness process, it may be necessary to help clients along through gentle reminders to focus on themselves and not on their partners. One husband I worked with summed up the importance of eventually "cleaning up his own side of the street" in saying to his wife "I now realize how much I was controlling and belittling you. I can see why a part of you wanted to get away from me and be with someone who treated you with more respect." He was able to acknowledge this, while still holding her completely responsible for how she chose to deal with her hurt, anger, and sense of loneliness.

The Overt Act of Forgiveness and Restoration of Love and Trust

While expressions of forgiveness may also occur throughout the process of forgiveness, they are particularly powerful when preceded by the work of the previous tasks. Overt forgiveness at this point can take many forms. For one betrayed spouse it occurred as he embraced his wife and verbally expressed for the first time, "I forgive you." For another, it was done through a note saying, "I would marry you again even after all we have been through." Helping the couple create meaningful rituals in which forgiveness can be expressed and received is often helpful at this point in therapy. The letters they started early on in therapy can be integrated at this point. Often, couples have a desire to renew vows.

The therapist can help a couple move toward greater degrees of relational trust through encouraging couple interactions that have not taken place since the affair was discovered. For one couple this was the resuming of their sexual relationship. For another, greater levels of trust became evident as she no longer felt inclined to check the computer for e-mails from his former online lover. The work of this task also includes celebrating his/her successes, wishing him/her well, and expressing love and support. I usually have clients write a separate letter of love and appreciation toward the end of their forgiveness journey, which they often report is the "corner" they needed to turn.

THE PROCESS OF APOLOGY

As stated previously, relational trust is most likely to be restored if the involved partner is actively working on his/her apology work as the forgiveness work of the betrayed partner is unfolding. Too often, the involved partner wants to help his/her partner heal, and yet is unsure about what to do beyond saying "I'm sorry," "I won't do it again," or "I hope you can forgive me somehow." The process of apology outlined in Table 2 helps him/her go beyond "I'm sorry" and to provide a format for taking complete responsibility for hurtful behavior, and then doing everything possible to make restitution and not repeat hurtful behavior.

Acknowledge What You Did to Hurt/Offend Him/Her

Much like the first task of the process of forgiveness, the work of disclosure and accountability can be more complex than it initially appears. Many involved partners want or need the therapist's help in navigating the fine-line between secret keeping and saying too much. The disclosure is most healing when it is honest, free of blame or excuse-making, and with sincere remorse. It also needs to include any specifics that clarify significant hurtful acts within the overall betrayal. Regarding how complete to make the disclosure, I often raise questions such as, "Is this information likely to come out later, and if so, will your partner feel betrayed that it wasn't shared from the start?" Or, "what would you be upset about if it were kept from you." To further clarify I will often tell clients to "explain that you did have intercourse, but not what positions you used or how long it lasted that one memorable night."

Learn How What You Did Impacted Him/Her and Express an Understanding of That Impact

The focus within this task is victim empathy. Betrayed partners usually want to know that their partners really understand how traumatic the betrayal was. The paradox, however, is that the offending partner is not likely to ever fully understand what it has been, is, and will be like to be in the betrayed partner's situation. Nevertheless, he/she should do all possible to "get it." While there are numerous ways of gaining this un-

TABLE 2. The Process of Apology

1. Acknowledge what you did to hurt/offend him/her.
2. Learn how what you did impacted him/her and express an understanding of that impact.
3. Make restitution where needed and possible
4. Learn how and why you did what you did, and share understanding with other person.
5. Identify and share your plan of action to not repeat hurtful behavior.
6. Overtly apologize and ask for forgiveness.
7. FOLLOW THROUGH!!

derstanding, the best source is undoubtedly the betrayed partner, him or herself.

Far too often, however, the involved partner either avoids asking questions which might lead to an expression of intense hurt or anger, or becomes defensive or inattentive in response. Therefore, encouraging the involved partner to sincerely ask about what the other is thinking or feeling, to read books describing the possible impact on the betrayed partner, or to participate in group therapy in which others talk about their experience of a partner's affair, can all be helpful means for increasing a sense of victim empathy. Experiential techniques can also be helpful, including inviting the involved partner to "stand in the other's shoes" by asking him/her to tell the story of the affair through the betrayed partner's perspective. Following this particular intervention, one client expressed being "amazed at how real it became after the first couple of questions." When these insights translate into greater degrees of remorse and expressions of understanding and empathy, healing is much more likely to occur. One helpful tool for the expression of victim empathy is the acronym "VUE," which stands for validation, understanding, and empathy. I encourage clients to "Do the VUE" as often, as deeply, and as sincerely as possible throughout the process of apology.

Make Restitution Where Needed and Possible

The main focus of restitution after an affair is, of course, on trust. Restitution of other losses may seem impossible, given the fact that what was taken, lost or "broken" is intangible. However, it is possible to reestablish a sense of fairness and balance within the relationship. For instance, one client who had spent a considerable amount of money on his affair (gifts, travel, hotels, etc.) decided to give up his season tickets to a local sports team, and dedicate the money instead for something they had both wanted to do as a couple but "couldn't afford." This act is different from the purchase of a ring or other gifts to "buy forgiveness or silence" from one's partner, as sometimes portrayed in the media.

Learn How and Why You Did What You Did, and Share Understanding with Other Person

It is important that the involved partner look beyond the obvious and determine both the methods and motives within the affair. The involved partner is often unaware of, or at least hesitant to acknowledge, the elaborate schemes used to cover up or justify the affair. One of my clients was an expert at convincing his wife that she was making a big deal out of nothing regarding his "friendship" with a colleague. Another had secret cell phone numbers and a credit card for which the statements were sent to a P.O. box. Another simply took advantage of her husband's regular business travel and would "forget her cell phone" while running various errands.

There are a lot of reasons why someone decides to have an affair, none of which are likely to make it seem acceptable to the betrayed partner. Therefore, in identifying the underlying motives for being unfaithful, it is critical that both partners understand that it is being done for the sake of accountability and the development of a safety plan, rather than to excuse or justify. One heterosexual client was particularly confused about why she ended up in a one year sexual relationship with her best friend of the same sex. Through the course of therapy she realized that she had a deeply embedded mistrust of men from childhood sexual abuse. It was in this "friendship turned sexual" that she had first been able to feel unguarded with her sexuality. She had always been aware of the abuse, but not of the impact. From this awareness, she determined that she needed to work through childhood trauma and learn to be more open with her husband.

Once a greater understanding of the methods and motives for the affair is gained, these insights can be shared with the betrayed partner. This process helps clarify the context in which the betrayal took place, helps him/her become less likely to see the infidelity as indicative of personal worth, and helps lay the groundwork for a comprehensive plan of action aimed at creating safety and fidelity in the relationship. As therapists, modeling ways in which insights can be shared without excuse-making can be helpful.

Identify and Share Your Plan of Action to Not Repeat Hurtful Behavior

As mentioned previously, an affair is often "crazymaking" for the betrayed partner due to the loss of consistency, predictability and safety. In an effort to re-establish some semblance of safety and determine if reconciliation makes sense, he/she usually asks "how are you going to make sure you never hurt me this way again?" Therefore, it is critical as therapists to help the involved partner change insight into action. Thus, for each "how" or "why" identified in the previous task, a "what now then" should follow. The more comprehensive the plan, the greater success he/she will have in not repeating hurtful behaviors and thus in restoring relational trust. The development of the involved partner's action plan and subsequent follow-through is central to the restoration of trust for most couples. For this reason, it is important to share and implement the plan of action and accountability as soon as possible, as it will likely become a barometer of sincerity and commitment to change.

Overtly Apologize and Ask for Forgiveness

Expressions of "I'm sorry" or "you didn't deserve this" hopefully have been made throughout the process of apology. Encouraging the involved partner to "say it again, and say it often," especially after the sincere work of previous tasks, is a simple yet effective therapeutic tool. Worthington and DiBlasio (1990) recommend couples have a "forgiveness session" in which each partner comes prepared to express apology or forgiveness. This can be an excellent time to integrate the sharing of the letters they began early in therapy. These and other rituals can be used to help the couple create positive experiences which can eventually overshadow those surrounding the affair. In a recent session, a client's simple, heart-felt, and tearful statement "will you please forgive me" following weeks of hard work in rebuilding trust with his wife was received by her with a long embrace and her own tears. We all knew they still had some rough times ahead, but they each expressed on many occasions that their relationship was ironically "much better than it was before the affair."

Follow Through!

For many betrayed spouses, the test of time is crucial. The broken promises and dishonesty that often accompany an ERA have left them focused on actions, not words. The on-going process of healing is difficult and relatively unpredictable. Therefore, it is important that as therapists we help the involved partner stay on track and not lose motivation despite occasional setbacks.

CONCLUSION

While many couples do not work toward reconciliation after an affair, a surprising number do. When appropriate, helping clients hang on to hope through this difficult journey is an important role played by marital therapists. As we lend our perspective about how healing *is* possible despite their sense of hopelessness, many couples are able to achieve relational growth well beyond what they ever thought possible. A comprehensive, mutual process of apology and forgiveness as outlined here can help provide the post-affair couple with the roadmap they need to find the healing they are seeking, at least in part, through therapy.

REFERENCES

Donnelly, D. (1966). *Putting forgiveness into practice.* Allen, TX: Argus Communications.

Enright, R. D., Santos, M., & Al-Mabuk, R. (1989). The adolescent as forgiver. *Journal of Adolescence, 12*, 95-110.

Hargrave, T. D. (1994). *Families and forgiveness: Healing the wounds in the intergenerational family.* New York, NY: Brunner/Mazel.

Hope, D. (1987). The healing paradox of forgiveness. *Psychotherapy, 24*, 240-244.

Rosenak, C. M., & Harnden, G. M. (1992). Forgiveness in the psychotherapeutic process: Clinical applications. *Journal of Psychology & Christianity, 11*, 188-197.

Simon, S., & Simon, S. (1990). *Forgiveness: How to make peace with your past and get on with your life.* New York, NY: Warner Books.

Smedes, L. B. (1983). Forgiving people who do not care. *Reformed Journal, 33*, 13-18.

Spring, J. A. (1997). *After the affair: Healing the pain and rebuilding trust when a partner has been unfaithful.* New York, NY: Harper Perennial.

Worthington, E. L., & DiBlasio, F. A. (1990). Promoting mutual forgiveness within the fractured relationship. *Psychotherapy, 27*, 219-223.

Split Self Affairs and Their Treatment

Emily M. Brown

SUMMARY. The Split Self Affair is a long-term serious relationship. The split being played out in the affair reflects an internal split between doing things "right" and the emotional self. Treatment for those involved centers on understanding the origins of the internal split and on reclaiming the neglected emotional self. Long term individual therapy is the treatment of choice, augmented by other modalities. *[Article copies available for a fee from The Haworth Document Delivery Service: 1-800-HAWORTH. E-mail address: <docdelivery@haworthpress.com> Website: <http://www.HaworthPress.com> © 2005 by The Haworth Press, Inc. All rights reserved.]*

KEYWORDS. Affair, infidelity, Split Self Affair, marriage, betrayed/betraying/betrayal, emotional self, internal split, "do it right," therapy, therapist, third party, betrayed spouse, betraying partner, individual therapy, couples therapy, group therapy, family therapy, emotions, feeling, rational self

The Split Self Affair is made for TV: it has romance, suspense, civility/refinement, and just the right amount of drama. The affair begins when a strong friendship evolves into a serious and enduring love affair.

Address correspondence to: Emily M. Brown, LCSW, 1600 Washington Blvd., Suite 702, Arlington, VA 22209.

[Haworth co-indexing entry note]: "Split Self Affairs and Their Treatment." Brown, Emily M. Co-published simultaneously in *Journal of Couple & Relationship Therapy* (The Haworth Press) Vol. 4, No. 2/3, 2005, pp. 55-69; and: *Handbook of the Clinical Treatment of Infidelity* (ed: Fred P. Piercy, Katherine M. Hertlein, and Joseph L. Wetchler) The Haworth Press, Inc., 2005, pp. 55-69. Single or multiple copies of this article are available for a fee from The Haworth Document Delivery Service [1-800-HAWORTH, 9:00 a.m. - 5:00 p.m. (EST). E-mail address: docdelivery@haworthpress.com].

The betraying partner, most often a man,[1] wants to leave his marriage to be with the third party, but does not, or does not leave for long. The betrayed spouse knows of her husband's affair, ruminates about it, but puts up with it hoping that he will come to his senses and want to be with her. Meanwhile, the third party is waiting for him to leave his marriage and is reminding him of his promises to do so. A stalemate ensues. The action on the part of the betraying partner consists of ending the affair with the intent to work on the marriage, followed by resuming the affair with the intent to end the marriage. Moving in and out is often a part of the action. The betrayed spouse and the third party play a waiting game, both tugging at the betraying partner with occasional well-mannered shots at each other.

The Split Self Affair presents an enigma to many therapists. Why are such bright, successful, and conscientious people having so much trouble doing the right thing (whatever that is)? What is keeping them so stuck? Understanding the dynamics underlying the Split Self Affair is the first step for therapists in working with either the Betraying Partner, the Betrayed Spouse, or the third party. Misunderstanding the meaning of these affairs leads to interventions that don't work such as urging the betrayed spouse to "kick him out," placing the primary focus on improving communication, using a couples format when individual therapy is needed, insisting that the affair end in order to continue therapy, or pushing the betraying partner to make a decision about the marriage. It also leads to frustration for the therapist.

The origins of the Split Self Affair lie in early childhood. Growing up in a situation that demands rationality and performance and that precludes paying attention to one's own emotions sets the stage. The split that is being played out in the affair reflects an internal split between doing things "right" and the emotional self. The specifics are different in different families. In some families "doing it right" means not attending to any emotional issues, or in other words, tuning out the emotional self and using only the rational self. In other families, performance is all. The children learn that coming out on top or winning is what is important, and that one's own emotions do not matter.

> *Dave, for example, grew up with a mother who was always hurt if Dave didn't do what she wanted him to do. Dave found it easiest to try to please her. When he didn't yield to his mother's neediness and instead did something that mattered to him, he paid for it emotionally with guilt at the hurt he caused his mother. Dave was in a double bind: he could caretake his mother and give up a piece of*

himself, or he could take care of himself and feel guilty. Dave coped by doing it right (caretaking his mother) most of the time, and hiding those activities that he thought his mother would react to with hurt. It is this kind of a bind that underlies the Split Self Affair.

Sometimes the demands to perform are self-imposed as a way of coping with profound neglect, or a crazy or dysfunctional family style. The child may decide to "do it right" as a way of trying to get needed attention, again tuning out the emotional self.

Steve's family situation was a bit different. His mother was an alcoholic whose word could not be trusted. His father was a much-loved person in their town whose work kept him busy and out of the house. The message Steve got from his parents' behavior was "You don't count." He coped by trying to do everything well so that he could show his parents that he was a good person and worth their attention. He attempted to rescue his mother from her alcohol addiction. He took care of his younger siblings as well as his mother. His parents didn't seem to notice his efforts but he got positive attention at school and from other adults in his small community. He chose a very demanding profession and has excelled at it. He married a woman who is a "good person"–she is not emotionally expressive but he wasn't looking for that–he'd had enough of emotional expression with his mother's drunken episodes.

Steve's affair was with a flamboyant, dishonest borderline who was much like his mother. Here was a second chance to "save his mother," and break the hold of the old message, "You don't count." As a bonus, Steve got some emotional intensity in his life.

In tuning out the emotional self, the individual is left with only the rational self. Thus one side of the split is the dominant rational side with a "do it right" approach; the other is the buried emotional self with needs that have not been met. It is important for therapists to understand the origins of this split and to realize that the rational "do it right" focus has been a matter of survival.

Meanwhile, the neglected emotional self lies dormant and largely unknown, waiting like Cinderella to be brought to life. A close friendship with someone who taps into this dormant emotional self is life-giving. The emotional vitality feels irresistible and the friendship evolves into an affair. The internal split is being played out but is externalized as a matter of choosing the right woman. It is useful to think of the affair as the unconscious recreation of a problem from childhood and an opportunity to resolve the underlying issue. The problem is not which partner to choose—it is the internal split.

The affair has opened the door to acknowledging the split. Healing the internal split is essential to resolving the situation. Until the rational and emotional selves come together and are owned, any decision about ending the marriage or the affair is likely to be reversed. Working with Split Selves looks deceptively easy at first. They are likeable people, their focus on working hard and doing it right often means professional success, they work hard in therapy (and they pay their therapist promptly), their conflict is low level, and they do a lot of thinking about their situation. Too much thinking! Staying rational is the kiss of death for them in therapy. Working with Split Selves requires persistent confrontation, a focus on the emotional, a strong hand in redirecting the work, and the ability to tolerate major ambivalence and behavioral flip-flops. Short term therapy will not work, although both the betrayed spouse and the third party want resolution now.

During the course of therapy, the male betraying partner will probably move out of the marital residence and move in with the third party, only to move home again a short time later, followed by another move out. This flip-flopping is symbolic of the Split Self's attempt to resolve the internal split by external means: specifically by choosing the "right" partner. Therapists need to avoid getting drawn into preventing the flip-flops, and keep the focus on the internal work. Females betraying partners are less apt to move out, usually because they have children at home.

COUPLES THERAPY

Some Split Selves present initially as a couple following discovery of the affair. Both spouses entered marriage with the idea that they would work hard and do marriage right. There may have been one or two Conflict Avoidance Affairs[2] in the past but they were glossed over. Little if any discussion transpired between the spouses about what had occurred or why, and the pain and guilt were pushed aside in an attempt to make the marriage work. The affair may have been as brief as a one night stand or have lasted for a few months, but the relationship with the third party was not a significant one. The Split Self Affair, however, is a serious and long-lasting relationship between the betraying partner and the third party. Attempts to end the affair fail, and the betrayed spouse's anger and obsession increases. They come for therapy when their efforts are not bearing fruit and they are feeling ground down by the dissension between them.

The stated goals of the betrayed spouse are to understand why the affair occurred and to get the marriage "back on track." However, she is focused on the affair and constantly questions her partner about all the details, interspersed with "how could you's." If she expresses any emotion it is anger, but the anger keeps her from paying attention to her deeper emotions such as pain, fear, or helplessness. The betraying partner wants help in dealing with his spouse's obsession with the affair. He feels guilty and tries to apologize and appease. He has been trying to answer the spouse's obsessive questions, sometimes with the full truth but often with less than the truth, the latter so as to "protect" the spouse from further hurt. Usually, the spouse knows when the response is not the full truth and badgers the betraying partner with more obsessive questions. Even when he is telling the whole truth, it is not enough. Obsession may seem like an expression of emotion because of the tone of voice or the body language but it is really rumination, a behavior that is in the rational realm and not the emotional. You might think of it as an irrational rational process.

The initial work is helping the betrayed spouse experience the basic emotions that underlie her obsession with the affair and to share those emotions with the betraying partner. It is important to elicit primary emotions such as pain, fear, and helplessness, and not settle for anger which is a secondary emotion. Experiencing one's primary emotions is grounding: It is a matter of experiencing the core self, rather than attacking the betrayer or endlessly ruminating about the affair. At the same time the betraying partner needs help from the therapist in being fully honest. These tasks dovetail: the pain expressed by the betrayed spouse evokes genuine remorse in the betraying partner rather than a defensive reaction. This brief emotional connection provides hope.

Many therapists insist that the affair end in order for therapy to continue.[3] The Split Self Affair is not going to end right away. Ending the affair would mean losing the connection to the newly found emotional self. To insist that it end prematurely pressures the betraying partner to resolve the ambivalence by flip-flopping between the marriage and the affair. Another eventuality is that the affair goes underground again. The affair will not end quickly because the betraying partner will continue to play out his split externally through the affair until the internal split is healed. Only then, when he has developed a strong emotional self, will he be able to end the affair for good.

If anyone insists the affair end, it needs to be the betrayed spouse. However, she will not be able to do so with any conviction in the early phase of therapy because she does not want to lose her partner. If she reacts to the disclosure by telling him to get out, it is not necessarily because she wants him out but because she has been told by family, friends, or professionals that she should kick him out. In these cases, he will probably move in again before long. Later in therapy, after she has worked on healing her own split, she may decide not to put up with the situation and insist on a separation. Such a decision can be empowering.

And yes, in Split Self situations the betrayed spouse is usually split internally as well. For both spouses the internal split is best addressed in individual therapy. Many of these couples, however, are enmeshed. The enmeshment results from their "doing family right" approach. Using couples therapy to untangle some of the enmeshment is very helpful preparation for individual therapy. Keep in mind that this is not marriage counseling–this couple is not ready to commit to working on the marriage. They do need help in sorting out where they are and what their next steps are. Some couples work is also useful as an adjunct to individual therapy in helping the spouses learn to share their emerging emotional selves with each other and much later, to explore and make decisions about the marital relationship.

INDIVIDUAL THERAPY

Individual therapy needs to be the core treatment modality for Split Selves, ideally for each spouse. They will have fewer restraints on talking freely if they see separate therapists. Hopefully both therapists are directing their attention to healing the internal split. When one therapist is working in that direction and the other spouse's therapist is saying, "You shouldn't put up with that" (not "I wonder why you're putting up with that"), chances for the couple to make their own decisions about their relationship are reduced.

Working with the Betraying Partner

Many Split Selves choose individual therapy from the beginning, particularly betraying partners who are troubled by their own behavior. Most have told their spouse of the affair or the spouse has discovered it, although the full picture may not have been shared. If you are seeing the betraying partner only, telling the spouse the truth can come later. This is not the case when working with a couple.[4]

Initially, the stated goal of the betraying partner is to get help in deciding which partner to choose: the spouse or the third party. This can be reframed as an internal split that is being played out externally. The work to be done consists of:

- identifying how it came to be that the rational and the emotional selves are mutually exclusive,
- healing the split so that the emotional and the rational selves are integrated.

It is only toward the end of this process that a solid decision about the marital relationship can be made.

The early work focuses on helping the individual learn about his or her emotional self, a self that is largely unknown. When asked, "What are you feeling right now?" the Split Self typically will give the therapist a "report" on what he has thought or observed, what he has made of his observations, and a few words about what he felt at some point in the past. Split Selves have great difficulty tuning in to what they are feeling at the moment, and need the therapist's help in learning how to do so.

You might start with the question: "What are you feeling right now?" When the typical answers emerge, ask, "What is going on emotionally inside you this very minute?" Then pause, giving the client some space to look inside. The client probably will not know. In that case, begin guiding the person, asking what he is experiencing in his physical self at the moment, and then pausing again. If he can't identify anything physical, ask whether he is experiencing any tension or discomfort in any part of his body. Help him identify the sensation and the specific location of the sensation. Once he is able to do so, ask what emotions are connected to that physical sensation.

In our first session, Matt alternated between obsessing about his wife's affair and covering his emotions with cheery bravado. I asked him what he was feeling. When he had difficulty with that question I shifted to asking about his physical self. Matt was finally able to say that he felt tense in his chest and on the sides of his face. At this point, his manner quieted down. I asked him to let himself feel that tension for a minute or so without thinking about how to fix it or trying to get rid of it. When his face changed after a minute,

I asked what emotion he was experiencing–what was the emotion that was underneath the tension in his body. He replied that it felt like when his father died. I asked how he had felt then. Matt said he felt like he had a hole in his body. He was able to move from there to saying he felt empty and afraid. I asked him to again just stay with what he was feeling, and he did so. As these emotions began to ebb away, I told him, "Feelings are like thoughts–they ebb and flow. Give them their space, and when they start going away, let them go." Before we ended I suggested that when Matt feels his chest or face are tight or finds himself obsessing about his wife's affair, that he tune in again to his physical self and then to his emotions. Because Split Selves are so perfectionistic, I also told him that he won't do it perfectly, so don't get down on himself, just get back on the track of paying attention to what he is feeling.

Tuning in to one's underlying emotions is grounding. It helps the person know where he is and enables him to avoid spinning out in response to other people's actions. It takes time and effort for Split Selves to make a habit of tuning into their emotions. Thus, this is the focus of much of the early work with Split Selves. You must constantly ask what the person is feeling and cut short the "reports," analyses, and other digressions. Parallel with the focus on emotions is identifying the origins of the internal split between doing things right and attending to self. Getting a detailed family history makes it possible to pinpoint how this pattern developed and why it was needed. The history needs to include what the client was feeling when key events occurred or in the face of repeated dysfunctional behavior in the household, and how he learned to cope with those difficult or traumatic situations. When family information is lacking or fragmented, discussions with other family members can fill in gaps. Family members often, although not always, feel honored to be asked to share their knowledge about the family and the past. Some family members are even willing to be taped. You and client can discuss who to talk to, what questions to ask, and how to ask in a way designed to put the family member at ease to the extent possible. The Split Self may need time to mull this over before moving ahead, so as to anticipate and prepare for the possible consequences of venturing into uncharted territory.

As the Split Self becomes more adept at identifying his emotions, it becomes possible for him to start working on being honest, first with himself, and then with others. Most Split Selves are deeply troubled by their dishonesty, and many recognize themselves that honesty is their next battleground. Once stated as a goal by the client, you need to keep on eye on how it is going. If the client does not volunteer the information, inquire about it. Being honest, combined with paying attention to one's emotions, opens the door to a different level of communication. Now there is the possibility of saying what one really feels, despite the risk of a negative response. This wasn't feasible early in life. The ability to voice one's emotions, combined with emotional honesty, makes in-depth conversation possible. This is the point at which the betraying partner can begin to talk honestly about the affair with his spouse.

The Split Self usually comes to the point where he decides to put the affair on hold. It is not that the emotional attachment is cut, but the Split Self has decided that he needs time and space to explore his emotional self by himself. This is not a flip-flop–the flip-flop is about choosing the right partner. The Split Self knows that the third party may no longer be there if he eventually decides to end his marriage. During this period, Split Selves can benefit from living alone. This helps end co-dependent behavior and facilitates time alone for exploring the self.

At first, being alone is hard to handle. Male Split Selves often have no close friends. A lifetime spent doing things right, both at home and at work, left little time for friendships. Men in our society are not encouraged to develop close friendships with other men. The third party has been the only "friend." There are choices to be made about how to use the "alone time." Will time be spent with the spouse? With the third party? Will he watch the movie or the game on TV? Will he just go to bed and sleep? You can encourage the Split Self to monitor the choices he makes, noting what he is feeling, what he is thinking, what he decides to do, and how it works out. With that self-monitoring, the Split Self gradually moves to a deeper examination of each choice that he makes. It is here that he begins to explore what he wants to do with his free time. Typically, he encounters some inner struggles between doing what he wants and doing something else because it would be the right thing to do. However, at this point he at least knows what he wants to do. Examples of what Split Selves have chosen are oil painting, sailing, making friends to hang out with, writing, and hiking. The possibilities are limitless. As the Split Self makes choices, he starts building a life. He also starts enjoying life more and moves away from the old "do it right" path so that there is a balance between attending to his responsibilities and paying attention to how he feels and what he wants. As with all therapy clients, the Split Self will make some choices that do not serve him well. However, by the time he is consciously making choices, he can learn from them. Your role is to facilitate examination of his choices, good and bad, elicit his evaluation of himself, help him trouble-shoot problem areas, and offer encouragement for continuing his work. Split Selves can expect that it will take a minimum of two years of therapy and often substantially longer to heal the split and become a whole person. Not everyone is willing to make this big an investment, but it is almost impossible to resolve these issues without therapy.

Working with the Betrayed Spouse

When the betrayed spouse first comes to therapy, she is fighting her grief. She has been dealt a significant ego wound and has learned that her marriage is not as she thought it was. The ground feels so shaky that she protects herself by obsessing about his affair–if she could only understand she could do something. In order to deal with her grief, she will need to get to the emotions she has been avoiding by obsessing about his affair: usually pain, fear, and/or helplessness. This is done through the same process described in the earlier section on couples work. When she is in touch with her pain, she may be reluctant to share it with her husband for fear of being too vulnerable. He would probably find it hard to hear and would try to appease or apologize so as to avoid it. Thus, it is important for you to hear her pain and validate it. Urging her to move beyond the obsession or telling her to see an attorney or "kick him out" will not help. She almost always wants the marriage to continue. Whether that is possible will not be known for a long time.

You need to help the betrayed spouse focus on herself in the present, not in the past or the future. Depression is common, so evaluating for this is essential. Medication, as well as talk therapy, may be in order. Just as for the betraying partner, a detailed family history is needed in order to identify the origins of her issues, including how her rational and emotional selves became split. Parallel to that work, you can help her learn to pay attention and give voice to her emotional self, thereby facilitating a gradual integration of her emotional and rational selves. As soon as she is able to access her emotions, grief work–grief for the loss of her marriage as she knew it–can be productive.

When the betrayed spouse's obsession is largely unabated after the first four to six months of therapy, developing an extensively detailed genogram can be helpful. Instead of doing it on paper, use a large whiteboard so that all the information is right in front of her. Later, transfer the information to paper and give copies to her (and possibly a copy for her spouse too) so that she can give further thought outside the session to what the family dynamics have meant for her. Usually the genogram shows a history of repeated abandonments, losses, and betrayals, more than was admitted in the initial history taking. You can then help the betrayed spouse work through the old issues that parallel the current situation or impede addressing it. For example, some betrayed spouses are in denial about the pain of their childhood, and their obsession is an attempt to avoid or to make palatable the reality of the affair.

Other than continuing to obsess about her husband's affair, the betrayed spouse's biggest danger is thinking that because she didn't have the affair, she has little or no work to do on herself. Actually, she may have more work to do–she is the one who has been reluctant to rock the marital boat. You can help her understand how she contributed to making enough room in the marriage for an affair–how and why she learned the behavior patterns that helped set the stage for an affair. She will not like looking at this, although at some level she knows she had some part in setting the stage. However, understanding her role makes it easier for her to work on her issues. If both spouses do the work of healing their own internal split, there is a chance for the couple to develop an emotionally satisfying marriage.

End Phase of Individual Therapy

The final phase of individual therapy for Split Selves has to do with getting closure on the affair, and making decisions about the marriage. It is also the time for the betraying partner to make a genuine apology and ask for forgiveness. You can initiate a discussion with your client about the need to talk through unfinished business with the other spouse. You can help them do so in a session with you, with both therapists, or if they choose, by themselves.

If both spouses have done extensive individual work and think they might want to work on the marriage, you might consider some conjoint sessions. Alternatively, you might refer the spouses to another therapist for couples work. If a decision has already been made by either spouse to end the marriage, a few sessions with either or both therapists to address unfinished business and gain closure can be useful. By this time, however, some couples are able to talk well together even though their marriage is ending.

If only one spouse has worked on healing the internal split, chances for the marriage are very poor–the very growth that is positive for the individual often means outgrowing the other spouse. When the decision to separate is one-sided, it is generally made by the spouse who has dealt with his or her issues. His grief is not so sharp because the ending has been in sight for quite a while. Sadness becomes the dominant emotion at this point, sometimes accompanied by an undercurrent of guilt that goes back to the "do family right" beliefs of the past. An important task for you is helping your client surface such guilt and resolve it. The practical issues of ending also need attention. You can help your client develop a plan for ending the marriage in as amicable a way as possible. Making good referrals to competent divorce mediators, attorneys, and other professionals needs to be part of the planning process.

Some betrayed spouses only arrive at your door after the betraying partner has decided to end the marriage. You will need to focus on much the same work described earlier: dealing with depression, understanding how she learned the behavior patterns that are not working, and reclaiming the emotional self. In addition, you will need to help her with extensive grief work. When ready, you can help her prepare to talk with her former spouse about their relationship and its demise. You might suggest that she invite him in for a session or two in order to help her gain closure. Alternatively, she can meet with him by herself. She too, needs to request forgiveness for her contribution to setting the stage for an affair. If her former spouse is not available, you can help her gain closure in other ways, such as writing him a letter, one that may or may not be sent.

A betraying partner who has ended his marriage may decide to contact the third party about resuming that relationship. Sometimes it becomes clear that he has outgrown the third party. In other cases the relationship with the third party has promise. Whatever the situation, remarrying before the internal split is healed, or shortly after the marriage has ended is problematic. However, Split Selves who have done their work are usually in no rush to remarry. If they are in a rush, you need to question whether the work is really finished.

Split Selves who resolve their issues feel much more comfortable with themselves than ever before. They also are able to connect with other people in a way that was never possible. Some remark on the fact that they have become a "Grown-up."

GROUP THERAPY

The Split Self betraying partner usually does not know that others are in the same situation. Their professional success often contributes to a reluctance to discuss personal issues with work associates. When the third party is a work associate, as is commonly the case, such a discussion is viewed as out of the question. Shame also contributes to maintaining silence with work associates and friends. Friends tend to be few, because "doing it right" has meant working hard, often to the exclusion of having friends or fun.

Group therapy can begin to break down the barriers to discussion of personal and emotional issues. It is easier to see the dynamics in others than to see them in one's self. And it is very hard for an individual to hide his issues from others in the group because they know the script–they are living it too. Such a group can be periodic, time-limited, or weekly and ongoing, but it should supplement rather than replace individual therapy.

The periodic group serves the Split Self well. The group should be limited to betraying partners, male and female, who are able to access their emotions, at least to some extent. It can be started as a single two hour session with the stated goal of talking to others in a similar situation. Confidentiality is established at the beginning of the first session. By sharing their situation and their struggles, members give and gain support. Toward the end of the first session, you can ask if they would like to meet again, and if so, in what time frame. Monthly is usually the choice and a two hour session allows them to dig into issues with each other when they meet.

Another type of group is the psycho-educational group for betrayed spouses (including other affair types), again male and female. In leading such a group, you need to ensure that the focus is on healing and not on being victimized. Acknowledge pain but when self-pity or blame comes up, redirect the energy to more productive channels.

FAMILY THERAPY

Family therapy with Split Selves is sometimes a useful adjunct to individual therapy. Children who are worried or are acting out may benefit from one or more family sessions. Family can be constituted in various ways, as indicated in the following examples.

Lorraine's husband had moved out six months ago when she first came for therapy. She was depressed and despairing. Her grown children were worried. A family session was scheduled for her and her children. They wanted me to know just how worried they were. She had always been strong and now she was coming apart at the seams. Part of their agenda was to check me out as well—was I someone who could help their mother? Lorraine and I reassured the children that although Lorraine was depressed and hurting, she was not suicidal and not in danger. We discussed what is normal in this situation, and they seemed to feel reassured that their mother was in good hands.

Beth and Frank were still living together along with two teenagers, a son and a daughter, who knew about their father's long-term affair. The family was one that avoided anger and conflict. The daughter began acting out, rarely speaking to her father, and when she did speak she made scathing comments about his behavior. In a family session with all four, in which I spent some time with the daughter by herself, it came out that since Mom didn't stand up for herself with Dad, the daughter was stepping in for Mom. The daughter and I talked about my role being one of helping Mom learn to fight like a tiger. After that session the daughter's behavior with Dad started to soften.

THOUGHTS ON CLOSING

Therapists can expect to see more Split Selves affairs in future years. We are currently raising a generation of Split Selves. The pressure on children today to perform, to succeed, and to win, combined with restrictions on their opportunities to explore what interests them, are important elements in creating an internal split between doing things right and the emotional self, between thinking and feeling. In working with families and family members, therapists have a very significant role to play in helping parents develop realistic expectations for their children, while encouraging their children's sense of self, especially the emotional self.

NOTES

1. The Split Self Affair used to be a man's affair. That has changed somewhat, but more men than women are still the betraying partner in these affairs. Thus, in the interest of readability, I have used "he" in referring to the betraying partner and "she" for the betrayed spouse. Gender differences are noted in the text or in endnotes.

2. See Chapter 2, *Types of Affairs and their Messages*, in Brown, Emily M., *Patterns of Infidelity and Their Treatment*, Second Edition (2001). New York: Brunner/Routledge.

3. In the training on addressing affairs that I offer to therapists, many have declared that they will not work with a couple if the betraying partner does not end his affair.

4. The therapeutic process is blocked when the couples' therapist colludes with the betraying partner to keep the secret of the affair from the betrayed spouse. When the affair is discovered, as will probably happen, the betrayed spouse will experience the therapist's behavior as another betrayal.

Marital Infidelity:
The Effects of Delayed
Traumatic Reaction

Don-David Lusterman

SUMMARY. This paper describes the usual course of discovered marital infidelity and its predictable posttraumatic reaction. It contrasts this phenomenon with situations in which the initial reaction to discovery is suppressed, leading to a delayed traumatic reaction. It concludes with suggestions for the treatment of a delayed traumatic reaction, and suggestions designed to sensitize therapists to the possibility of a suppressed reaction to marital infidelity as a possible underlying issue in individual or couples therapy. *[Article copies available for a fee from The Haworth Document Delivery Service: 1-800-HAWORTH. E-mail address: <docdelivery@haworthpress.com> Website: <http://www.HaworthPress.com> © 2005 by The Haworth Press, Inc. All rights reserved.]*

KEYWORDS. Marital infidelity, extramarital affairs, delayed traumatic reaction, couples therapy, induced memory

---

Don-David Lusterman, PhD, is a psychologist in private practice, specializing in Marriage and Family Therapy.

Address correspondence to: Don-David Lusterman, PhD, 856 McKinley Street, Baldwin, NY 11510 (E-mail: PSY95@aol.com).

[Haworth co-indexing entry note]: "Marital Infidelity: The Effects of Delayed Traumatic Reaction." Lusterman, Don-David. Co-published simultaneously in *Journal of Couple & Relationship Therapy* (The Haworth Press) Vol. 4, No. 2/3, 2005, pp. 71-81; and: *Handbook of the Clinical Treatment of Infidelity* (ed: Fred P. Piercy, Katherine M. Hertlein, and Joseph L. Wetchler) The Haworth Press, Inc., 2005, pp. 71-81. Single or multiple copies of this article are available for a fee from The Haworth Document Delivery Service [1-800-HAWORTH, 9:00 a.m. - 5:00 p.m. (EST). E-mail address: docdelivery@haworthpress.com].

doi:10.1300/J398v04n02_07

INTRODUCTION

The initial reaction to the discovery of infidelity is almost invariably a shattering experience for the discoverer. Most people feel at that moment that their marriage has ended. They often react in ways that shock themselves as well as their partners. This may include threats of suicide or homicide. A violent physical reaction by the discoverer is not uncommon. An almost predictable sequel to discovery is a posttraumatic reaction, characterized by flashbacks, numbness, and hyperalertness (Lusterman, 1989, 1995, 1998; Glass, 1997, 2003). Over the last thirty years I have treated close to a thousand cases in which infidelity played a significant role. Perhaps because I have treated such a large number of cases involving infidelity, I have become aware of a small percentage of people whose reaction occurs long after the discovery or strong suspicion that an infidelity has occurred. In order to understand the special circumstances that flow from a long-delayed reaction to a serious trauma to the marriage, it is necessary first to review the more usual course of behavior following discovery.

THE USUAL COURSE OF DISCOVERY

Most discoverers report that they have gone through some period of time during which they experienced a subliminal concern that infidelity was occurring. During this time they tend to feel anxious, irritable, and often depressed. Despite these feelings, they report that they cannot "put their finger" on what is bothering them. Many years ago a patient described the period preceding discovery as "cold rage," a term that most of my patients accept as an accurate description of what they have experienced. This period often serves the need of the unfaithful partner to feel that the infidelity is justifiable–after all, he or she reasons, who could live with a person who is behaving so miserably? The increasingly difficult behavior of the person who is edging towards discovery thus serves as an acceptable reason for the unfaithful behavior to persist or intensify. At a certain point, it becomes impossible for the spouse who continues to believe that there is a monogamous relationship to further deny the infidelity. Often this occurs as a function of a massive number of details coalescing. Occasionally, the unfaithful partner will spontaneously admit that there has been, or continues to be, an infidelity. More often, changes in the spouse's use of time or money, the reports of friends, or a communication from the affair partner are likely signs of infidelity. Almost invariably what follows is the explosive behavior described earlier. The term "hot rage" well describes this reaction. Most often (although not always), it is at this point that the couple presents for therapy.

The posttraumatic reaction generally sets in almost immediately following discovery. Although numbness may be present, there is invariably also a profound hyperalertness, and a great need to learn "the truth, and all the truth." The unfaithful partner is generally reluctant to give the necessary information, for a variety of reasons. These include a fear of the discoverer's reaction, the possibility of some subsequent legal action, and, very often, a wish to protect the affair partner, even if the affair has ended. The discovered partner may have created such a fabric of lies that it is impossible to remember them all, or may be so ashamed of certain actions that memory of them is genuinely suppressed.

It is comforting to most couples confronting the effects of discovered infidelity to know that the posttraumatic reaction to infidelity is normal, and not a pathological state. Armed with this awareness, the unfaithful partner can learn the skills necessary to begin the process of helping the discoverer to heal through empathic acceptance of the discoverer's persistent anger and unending questions. At the same time, the discoverer is encouraged, once it is clear that the unfaithful behavior is no longer occurring, to begin the process of a gradual letting go of the suspicion, fear, and hyperalertness that were indeed a necessary defense following discovery. Patients also find it comforting to know that, for the most part, the traumatic reaction gradually subsides as it becomes clear that the affair is over, and that the couple's relationship is improving. It is often helpful to couples waiting for the posttraumatic reaction to abate to be reminded that "time alone does not heal trauma, but *good* time does."

Unlike most traumatic events, where the trauma is well-publicized (such as hurricanes, fires, war-related events), infidelity, like rape, is often a well-guarded secret. Thus the societal and personal support that many traumatized people receive following "public" trauma is often not available to the discoverer of infidelity. This is both a plus and a minus during the course of treatment. An advantage of silence is that one is not barraged by the advice of well-meaning friends and family. Often such advice is profoundly colored by the experience and the value system of the helper, and only increases the person's doubts about the manner in which he or she is reacting to the affair. Discoverers often report that the conflicting advice they receive provides them with much confusion and little comfort. On the other hand, when the person who had been unfaithful is patient, supportive and nonjudgmental, the discoverer receives the support necessary to begin the process of healing. This in turn permits the couple to discuss fully the nature of the infidelity. The willingness of the unfaithful spouse to be open and honest in replying to the questions that plague the discoverer serves, ironically, as an antidote to the painful effects of the lying that is an inevitable accompaniment to infidelity. As these tasks are accomplished, the couple is able to reexamine the marriage that preceded the infidelity. This often leads to significant change in their relationship.

DELAYED REACTION TO DISCOVERY

DSM-IV describes delayed PTSD as "symptoms that either develop more than six months after the trauma or last six months or more." The concept of delayed stress reaction is discussed by Rothbaum and Foa (1993), who cast doubt on the "delayed" category of PTSD, as well as other subsidiary forms. MacFarlane (as cited in Rothbaum and Foa, 1993) holds that "the definition of acute, delayed-onset and chronic PTSDs . . . may be an arbitrary generalization based on clinical experience." This chapter will present a number of clinical examples of delayed PTSD which represent a distinct clinical picture that is different in its nature from a rapid response to trauma, and requires different treatment. Much of science derives its inspiration from clinical observation, and often provides testable hypotheses. Certainly, controlled studies of these clinical observations are welcome.

The following case was my first experience with a long-delayed reaction and its consequences: Bill and Jennifer consulted with me concerning some problems they were experiencing with their eldest daughter, who was then 12-years-old. The couple also had two sons, aged eight and six. The case seemed simple enough. They had recently moved, and Jessica, who was just entering puberty, was disappointed and angry with her parents because the move necessitated a change of school districts, and the loss of much of her friendship network. Her parents were most cooperative. They made arrangements for sleepovers and other social events, and learned to listen more empathically to Jessica's struggles. It was not long before she began to adjust to her new situation.

At one session Bill had expressed some annoyance with Jessica's secrecy. "She's just like her mother," he said, with a little smile that seemed to indicate that it was nothing important. Jennifer said she felt offended, Bill apologized, and attention turned again to Jessica's secrecy, mostly about her increasing interest in some of the boys that she was meeting at her new school. Jennifer explained that there were some things that were more "mother and daughter" issues and that Jessica might feel a bit uncomfortable sharing these thoughts with her father. Jessica added: "After all, Dad, you *are* a guy." With good support, and much opportunity for Jessica to express her feelings, she soon felt considerably better, and therapy ended.

About five years later I received a panicked call from Jennifer. "You were so helpful about Jessica, so I am turning to you again. Bill has been acting really crazy. I haven't been able to get through to him all, but I finally convinced him that we should come in together." When they arrived for their first session, I barely recognized Bill. Never a heavy person, he had lost considerable weight. His face seemed drawn. His eyes were bloodshot, and he looked straight ahead, at no one in particular, but wide-eyed, and with an intense and unblinking stare. As he talked, he seemed to be containing so much rage that he could look at nothing but the wall. "This isn't about me. The problem is Jennifer, and I am not at all sure that the marriage can go on if she can't be honest with me." Inquiry revealed Bill's vague, unsupported suspicion that Jennifer was having what he called "a flaming affair." Jennifer vehemently denied this.

Of course, the possibility that it was true required some investigation. A session was arranged for Jennifer alone. The usual assurance was given to Bill and Jennifer (Lusterman, 1995) that anything that either of them said at an individual session would be respected by me as a confidence, but that, of course, what I learned would help me to determine the best mode of treatment. After considerable probing, I was convinced that there was no affair going on. At the session's conclusion, she began to cry, and indicated again her desperate concern for his well-being. "He's not going to work, he's angry with me and the children all the time. He barely eats, but he's started drinking beer, which he never did. He's just not his usual, sweet self. Maybe he needs hospitalization?"

For several months there was no progress at all. Jennifer remained convinced that he was in a serious "breakdown." Every effort she made to be empathic and helpful was greeted with Bill's ever-increasing suspicions. He demanded that she be accessible by phone every minute of the day. The slightest deviation from this plan enraged him. A psychiatric consult was arranged, with no dramatic results. A tranquilizer was recommended, but was not helpful. Therapy was at an impasse, and I had no idea what to do next. I explained my dilemma to the couple, and suggested that we take a few weeks off. "You came to me for change," I added, "but it's not happening."

When they returned, Bill's attacks on Jennifer had reached an even higher pitch. As the session continued, he began to pace the room, fists clenched. As he sat down he announced: "I found some pictures, and now I know what happened." He reached beneath his chair to place the attaché case that he had come with on his knees. It was crammed with pictures and documents. As he poured through the pictures, he described a process of detection over the past two weeks. "I looked at the invitation list to our wedding, and I saw the name of the guy you went with before we married. Then I realized that, several times in the six months before the wedding, you would disappear. It gave me a funny feeling that something was going on between you and this guy, but I guess I squelched it. Then I looked at wedding pictures. There you are–see–dancing with him, like you had stars in your eyes. Then I started putting together the times you disappeared. There were some snaps of you and him in a pile of photos, and I could see that you were with him, upstate, where I never went with you." Then he stood directly in front of her, waving the photographs, and shaking with rage. "Under my nose–you lied–you had an affair. I was so stupid. Admit it or it's all over."

Jennifer appeared dumbfounded. She was silent for what felt like an eternity. Then she spoke, so softly she could barely be heard. "What I did before we got married is my business. How stupid can you be? You can't have an affair *before* you're married. Affairs happen during marriage." "Jennifer," I asked, "are you saying that something happened between you and this person during your engagement?" "Yes," she replied, "but it was before we married, and I still wasn't sure about my decision. I had to know for certain if Bill or this guy was the one I should marry." "What defines an affair is its secrecy," I stated. "By that definition, it sounds as if Bill has reason to believe that you were acting dishonestly. Clearly, Bill saw your engagement as a commitment to a monogamous relationship, and therefore, your involvement with this other person is, for him, an act of infidelity."

There followed several painful sessions, during which Jennifer continued to maintain that it was none of Bill's business, until finally she confronted him. "Not only was I with him–I had sex with him, too. And I still think it's none of your business. After all, I made up my mind, and decided it was you and me, not me and him." Surprisingly, this admission seemed to calm Bill. I asked him if he was indeed feeling calmer. He agreed, but added that it wasn't because she had decided to stay with him, because there could have been a million reasons for that. No–what relieved him was that she finally admitted what had happened so many years ago. "So I'm not crazy, like you both thought." It surprised me to find that he had perceived a shared belief between Jennifer and me that he was "crazy." In retrospect, it is understandable that referring him to a psychiatrist would confirm that belief for him.

I have described elsewhere (Lusterman, 1998) what I call the "ticket of admission" back into marriage following an affair. It has two elements: admission and remorse. The discoverer needs desperately to know that the unfaithful person understands and regrets the pain that the infidelity has caused. For several sessions, Jennifer had evidenced no signs of remorse. During this time, his suspicions about her behavior during the marriage had intensified. He was convinced that she had been unfaithful many times. There were bitter fights, and persistent denials on her part. "Why would I believe you now, if it took all this time and detective work to get you to confess about what happened all those years ago?"

At that point, Jennifer requested a session alone. She told me that she couldn't lie and tell him that she didn't enjoy what happened between her and the other man. It would be a lie, and he would know it. "I think he wants me to tell him that I took no pleasure in what happened, but saying that would make him trust me even less," she said, "because he would know that I was lying." "I don't think your feelings about the pleasure that were part of the affair are the real issue," I replied. "Do you feel bad about pain that you caused Bill?" She assured me that she did, that she loved and respected Bill, and just wanted the Bill that she loved back again. I reminded her that the remorse that he needed to hear was about her realization that she had caused him such pain, if only she could bring herself to let him know. I pointed out how hard it had been for her to accept the fact that, from Bill's perspective, she had acted unfaithfully. Her refusal to acknowledge this had made him feel unheard, I pointed out, and had also intensified his current fears.

Over the next several meetings she was able to make clear to him that she could now accept his belief that she had acted unfaithfully, that she could understand why it shook him so badly, and felt genuine remorse for the pain that her actions had caused him. It was not long before his fears of a current infidelity dissipated. Following this, they were able to deal with other examples of what Bill saw as her dishonesty. Most of these concerned their children. Bill became aware that his often angry style of parenting caused Jennifer to protect them by withholding information from Bill. They both began to see how her protective stance and his "hardnosed" approach each amplified a pattern that neither wanted.

No evidence ever arose that supported his presenting problem–the fear that she was having an affair.

It was several years before they both agreed that they once again had an excellent marriage. As the initial trauma of discovery was assuaged in many ways, they were able to focus on other marital issues. Bill returned to work. The marriage has continued, and both agree, many years after therapy, that it is a good one.

DISCUSSION

During the many years since that first case, I have treated many other instances of long-delayed response to an earlier trauma of discovery. In some instances, as with this couple, the discovery did not take place until years afterward. In others, there was a mild and quickly submerged response. In still others, a therapist had mislabeled a healthy response to discovery as pathological, and caused it to go underground. The common element in these cases is the long delay before there is a full blown response to the unfaithful behaviors. In most cases of delayed response to trauma, the therapist is faced with a difficult challenge. Any therapeutic action that ignores the underlying cause further delays the support that the discoverer requires to begin to deal with the long-suppressed (or denied) reaction. For the most part, when couples present at or very shortly after discovery, the discoverer is already in "hot rage." With the benefit of much hindsight, I have come to realize that the long-dormant traumatic reaction may be analogous with the "cold rage" phase that usually precedes hot rage in cases of discovered infidelity. In treating delayed traumatic response, the therapist becomes aware, often with great difficulty, that the troubled partner never sensed the original infidelity, or behaved in an atypical manner when it was discovered.

My own error in the first case–the exploration of the possibility that Bill was experiencing some severe and perhaps delusional mental disorder, made him feel that both his therapist and his wife were conspiring against him. This is often the case when the therapist unsuspectingly blunders into the discovery of a delayed traumatic reaction. Therapists are well advised to carefully examine the presenting complaint, and if it appears insubstantial, to take a careful history of the marriage, dating back to the courtship and relationships that preceded the couple's first meeting. Often it is only this careful inquiry that creates an environment sufficiently safe that the original trauma may begin to surface.

While the case I have presented involves a husband who became suspicious of his wife's infidelity, this is not the only scenario. In another case, Betty, a woman then in her late 40s, discovered that her husband has been having an affair with her best friend. She told him that she was aware of what was going on and wanted it stopped immediately. Normally, this action would be followed by rage, and an enormous need to continue checking until she became certain that the affair was over. In this instance, within a short period of time, the marriage appeared to have returned to its prior state, with no excessive suspicion and no recriminations. Years later, the couple came to therapy because of her husband's concern with his wife's sudden depression and irritability. It was only through a careful examination of the early years of their marriage that the couple, for the first time, examined the impact of the event that had occurred so many years earlier. A review of her family of origin history focused on a situation that she had never talked about with her husband. When she was about twelve-years-old, her mother discovered that her father had been involved in several affairs. Her mother reacted with enormous rage, and it was not long before the marriage ended in a bitter divorce. Betty, the eldest of three, and the only daughter, had been very close with her father. Following the divorce, her mother moved to another state, and contact between the father and his children ceased. For the first time, Betty could understand why her initial reaction had been so bland. When she discovered her husband's affair, she could now see, the fear that her daughter, then just thirteen, might lose her father overwhelmed Betty. "I guess I just shut down, because I was so afraid of that possibility," Betty explained. Understanding this history, it was easier for this couple to understand how completely Betty had shut down. Only then was it possible for Betty to express her rage at her husband, and for the couple to begin their long-delayed recovery from the effects of his infidelity.

In another case, a recently married man unexpectedly returned home at midday because he was not feeling well. Hearing noise in the bedroom, he flung the door open, to find his wife and another man having intercourse. He was momentarily enraged, ordered the man to leave, and told his wife that this must never happen again. After a few days, the matter was dropped. Fifteen years later, the man announced to his wife that he was madly in love with another woman, and would like to separate in order to be sure that ending the marriage would be the proper decision. He agreed, however, to attend therapy with his wife, towards whom he felt, as he said, "no animosity." As therapy proceeded, little more was said about his passionate affair, and his wife was confused by his inability to talk about anything in the marriage or his personal life that might have precipitated the affair. After several sessions of fruitless examination of this question, he blandly wondered aloud at a therapy session: "I wonder if this might have anything to do with that time I found you in bed with that guy?" He reported that he has never thought about this before, but that something in the last few therapy sessions made him sense how vengeful he was feeling. I suggested that perhaps this was a long-delayed retaliatory affair. He looked quite amazed when this suggestion was offered, and sat quietly for a while. "That's incredible, but I think maybe you're right." It was suggested that he enter individual therapy, because he seemed so unable to express feelings about either the past or the present. As his ability to express his feelings improved, we were able to deal with issues in the marriage that he had never spoken about. As these were worked through, the affair ended.

In still another case, a woman who discovered her husband's lengthy affair with her best friend was told by their therapist that she was pathologically jealous, and that if she didn't stop her "inappropriate" behavior, she would undoubtedly do her marriage great harm. Ten years later her husband insisted that they begin couples therapy, because she was so depressed and irritable that the marriage was "in trouble," and might not survive if she couldn't be helped. A major element in this case was the review of the bind that the therapist had unwittingly created for this woman. Her husband, who at first felt relieved about the silencing of his wife's anger, began to see how, instead, it had simply numbed her into a state that froze their relationship for many years.

TREATMENT ISSUES

The suggestions that derive from this information may be of use in two very different situations. One, of course, is directed to the therapist who discovers a delayed traumatic reaction. The other is directed toward the therapist who is treating a person in the throes of discovery.

The therapist who treats a person in the throes of discovery will be most helpful to the discoverer if the trauma of discovery is accepted and respected. If the patient comes alone, reassurance should be given that this reaction is normal, acceptable, and if properly handled, time-limited. If at all possible, even if it seems evident that a divorce is inevitable, every attempt should be made to include the marital or relationship partner in at least some of the sessions. If the treating therapist is not trained in family and couples therapy, an appropriate referral should be made. If the family and couples therapist has not had training or workshops concerning the treatment of infidelity, an attempt should be made to find one who is.

The most important caveat that derives from an understanding of the phenomenon of delayed traumatic reaction is that one must be conscious of the possibility that a long-unprocessed infidelity may account for what otherwise appears to be unusual and perhaps pathological behavior on the part of one member of the couple. Clearly, if a patient has a long history of some form of pathology, the therapist must investigate the possibility that the current behavior is simply "more of same." In cases where the person's partner expresses great surprise about the behavior, and there is no evidence of a present infidelity, the therapist should be alerted to the possibility of a delayed traumatic reaction. It is at this point that a careful review of the couple's courtship, early marriage and relationships that preceded the marriage may suggest the possibility of an unprocessed infidelity. The clarity with which this inquiry is conducted may permit the traumatized partner to begin a process of introspection that leads to the exploration of such an event. The therapist is cautioned not to "induce" a memory, because there is the danger of inducing a false memory. All that the therapist can do is to create a safe therapeutic environment in which the issue may arise and, if it does, be explored.

REFERENCES

American Psychiatric Association. (1994). *Diagnostic and statistical manual of mental disorders (4th ed.).* Washington, DC: American Psychiatric Association.

Glass, S. (2003). *Not just friends: Protect your relationship from infidelity and heal the trauma of betrayal.* New York: The Free Press.

Glass, S.P., & Wright, T.L. (1997). Reconstructing marriages after the trauma of infidelity. In W.K. Halford & H.J. Markman (Eds.), *Clinical handbook of marriage and couples interventions.* New York: Wiley.

Lusterman, D-D. (1989). Marriage at the turning point. *The Family Therapy Networker.*

Lusterman, D-D. (1995). Treating marital infidelity. In Mikesell, R.H., Lusterman, D-D., & McDaniel, S. (Eds.), *Integrating family therapy: Handbook of family psychology and systems theory.* Washington DC: American Psychological Association.

Lusterman, D-D. (1998). *Infidelity: A survival guide.* Oakland, CA: New Harbinger Publications, Inc.

Rothbaum, B.O., & Foa, E.B. (1993). Subtypes of posttraumatic stress disorder and duration of symptoms, in Davidson, J.R. & Foa, E.B. (Eds.), *Posttraumatic stress disorder: DSM-IV and beyond.* Washington DC: American Psychiatric Press, Inc.

"Accusatory Suffering" in the Offended Spouse

Frank J. Stalfa, Jr.
Catherine A. Hastings

SUMMARY. In this paper we describe the syndrome known as "accusatory suffering" as a dynamic in the treatment of marital infidelity. We also provide diagnostic criteria and a description of the effects of accusatory suffering in the course of therapy. A sample case is presented to explore therapeutic approaches. Recommendations are made for possible therapeutic initiatives that may enable couples to move beyond the impasse created by this type of defensive reaction. *[Article copies available for a fee from The Haworth Document Delivery Service: 1-800-HAWORTH. E-mail address: <docdelivery@haworthpress.com> Website: <http://www.HaworthPress.com> © 2005 by The Haworth Press, Inc. All rights reserved.]*

Frank J. Stalfa, Jr., DMin, is Pastoral Therapist, Samaritan Counseling Center of Lancaster County. He is Associate Professor of Pastoral Theology and Counseling, Lancaster Theological Seminary, Lancaster, PA, a Diplomate of the American Psychotherapy Association, a National Board Certified and Licensed Professional Counselor, and a member of the Pennsylvania Counselor's Association.

Catherine A. Hastings, PhD, is Marriage and Family Therapist, Samaritan Counseling Center of Lancaster County where she co-directs the Couple's Institute. She is a Clinical Member and Approved Supervisor in the American Association of Marriage and Family Therapy, and is a Licensed Marriage and Family Therapist in Pennsylvania.

[Haworth co-indexing entry note]: "'Accusatory Suffering' in the Offended Spouse." Stalfa Jr., Frank J., and Catherine A. Hastings. Co-published simultaneously in *Journal of Couple & Relationship Therapy* (The Haworth Press) Vol. 4, No. 2/3, 2005, pp. 83-90; and: *Handbook of the Clinical Treatment of Infidelity* (ed: Fred P. Piercy, Katherine M. Hertlein, and Joseph L. Wetchler) The Haworth Press, Inc., 2005, pp. 83-90. Single or multiple copies of this article are available for a fee from The Haworth Document Delivery Service [1-800-HAWORTH, 9:00 a.m. - 5:00 p.m. (EST). E-mail address: docdelivery@haworthpress.com].

KEYWORDS. Accusatory suffering, infidelity, adultery

Few couples are prepared for the emotional volatility of infidelity. Once the affair is revealed, both spouses confront intense reactions that go well beyond the familiar variations of anger and guilt. Most clinicians recognize the legitimacy of the offended spouse's feelings of victimization, and strive to honor the pain he or she feels as a result. In the initial stages of therapy, the angry disillusionment of the offended spouse is often so prominent that it becomes the necessary focus of attention.

In most cases, as the therapist encourages the offended spouse to vent, confront and inquire while the offending spouse listens, explains and accepts responsibility for the affair, the intensity of legitimate outrage lessens. The offender's sincere expression of remorse and desire to reestablish trust provides a basis for moving beyond the event that originally caused the pain. The couple may now look more deeply at the symptomatic significance of the affair itself. This is a treasured moment in the therapeutic process, a turning point we hope for, but too seldom achieve: the potential for the affair to serve as a catalyst for the renewal of the marriage.

There are many forces at work that serve to prevent couples using the affair to "grow" the marriage. One dynamic that most of us have confronted is "accusatory suffering," a term coined by Seagull and Seagull (1991), to mean "a necessity to suffer and create a living memorial to the infidelity." In the *AAMFT Clinical Update on Infidelity,* Glass (2000) defines accusatory suffering as:

> . . . an unconscious idea that full recovery would exonerate the perpetrator from blame. The betrayed spouse fears that doing too well would invalidate the pain and suffering they experienced–causing their partner to minimize the consequences of their actions and be unfaithful again.

As with most symptomatic responses to the pain of infidelity, accusatory suffering can be acute or chronic; it may represent a phase in the process of healing or become a permanent and entrenched position that effectively sabotages any further progress. It is this most extreme form that we will explore in this essay. First, we will expand the description of how accusatory suffering presents itself and then examine the treatment of this process through a case study.

The above-mentioned definition of accusatory suffering tells us a great deal about its function, both intra-psychically and interpersonally. We are safe to assume that as an unconscious defense against further pain, it may well have its origins in earlier experiences of loss and betrayal in the client's family of origin. In some cases it may be connected to more recent and actual betrayals in former relationships or even prior infidelities in the current marriage. Perhaps this is why in its most extreme form it has the resonance of post-traumatic stress disorder, suggesting that an earlier wound has been reactivated. In our experience, the most severe manifestation of this syndrome has the following characteristics: (1) the offended spouse is obsessionally focused on the profound violation of personal dignity resulting from the affair; (2) no apology or restitution, however heartfelt on the part of the offending spouse, suffices to mollify the offended spouse's anguish and may, indeed, elicit even more scornful denunciation; (3) the amount of time and effort expended in validating the offended spouse's pain–by offending spouse or therapist–does little to reduce its intensity; (4) any attempt to focus directly on the affair evokes an immediate and inexhaustible tirade from the offended spouse as though it is being relived from the initial moment of discovery; and perhaps, most important, (5) the vengeful rage of the offended spouse is *not characteristic* of her or his usual manner of dealing with marital discord. This last criterion is important. Certainly we might expect some spouses with explosive temperaments, borderline traits or tendencies toward pathological jealousy to react in extreme ways. However, offended spouses often experience true accusatory suffering as ego-dystonic–it doesn't fit how they see themselves. They feel they are in the grip of an irrational force they cannot control. They want to know how they can get beyond it and are honestly mystified by the power it has to override their better intentions. Most poignantly, it is as though they are partially aware of the inherent irrationality of their rage and its counter-productive consequences. They see how it serves to undermine their own desire to improve the marriage and yet can do nothing to change it. In this terrible dilemma, they ask us questions we cannot answer.

In order to respect fully the power of this syndrome, we must understand the belief system that generates its deep conviction. The offended partner is terrified of being made to look foolish again. She or he believes that one betrayal signifies a likely past affair or subsequent one. This symptom seems designed to resolve the conundrum of how to prevent a future betrayal, yet hold on to the marriage. It is as though the offended client is saying: "If I can convince you that what you did is

inconsolable for me, you will not dare to do it again and–most importantly–my pain will continue to chastise and discipline you and therefore confer on me some protection from another humiliation." This
seems to be the strategic intention behind unending accusatory suffering. The offending partner, however, is left with a sense that his or her
trustworthiness can never be re-established. This spouse is "on notice"
that any suspicious behavior may reactivate the original pain. The offending spouse, perhaps out of guilt, accepts this arrangement to maintain the fragile stability of the marriage. The two of them remain locked
in an untenable but seemingly necessary stalemate.

The resulting stalemate can last for a long time. In our experience, the
offended spouse is the only one who can change the process in one direction or another. She or he either leaves the marriage because trust is
terminally lost or agrees to work on the accusatory suffering as a
changeable manifestation of the pain of betrayal. However reasonable
accusatory suffering may seem, it also creates problems. Yet, it feeds on
one powerful dynamic: If the offended spouse takes responsibility for
how the accusatory suffering undermines progress, he or she is also
likely to feel that this syndrome–now perceived as a kind of diagnosis–has become the real issue, not the original affair. In one of the more
spectacular paradoxes of this dilemma, the offended spouse feels that
she or he is now the offending rather than the offended spouse. Their
roles and accountabilities have been reversed. Now the offending
spouse is the "victim" of the offended spouse's inability to "get over"
the affair. The therapist is frequently caught in an untenable position.
By trying to identify the countervailing influence of accusatory suffering, there is the perception that the therapist is now over-identifying
with the offending spouse. When the therapist tries once more to understand and validate the offended spouse's position by emphasizing a
need for greater empathy, the therapist is likely to hear the offending
spouse say, "Nothing is enough." If the therapist shifts to a position of
helping the unfaithful spouse set limits on what is acceptable in the form
of attacks for past infidelity and predictions of future betrayals, then the
offended spouse responds with even more intensified reactions. These
seem to be characteristic double binds inherent in this syndrome and
pose quite a challenge for the therapist and the couple. The resulting
stalemate threatens to bring therapeutic progress to an end. However,
the therapist has several options. They include:

• Go back to the original issue of betrayal to see if important pieces
  of information or emotional meaning have been overlooked.

- Trace related experiences of broken trust and disillusionment in the marital history to see if they are clouding the issue.
- Deal with the impact of the betrayal on the offended spouse's self-esteem, perhaps exploring family-of-origin dynamics.
- Focus on the offending spouse's lack of demonstrable remorse. Is he or she missing opportunities to rebuild trust? Is there a recognition that the affair will always be part of their history as a couple?

A CASE HISTORY

So far, we have established that accusatory suffering is, by its very nature, both irrational and strategic. Its tortured logic tries to resolve a paradoxical dilemma: how can the offended spouse simultaneously punish the offending spouse and, at the same time, protect the marriage against future betrayal? The following case illustrates some of the most potent dynamics in this syndrome without resolving the problem completely. Because it is a case still in progress, we will point to facets of the problem and *possible* therapeutic responses, rather than solutions.

"Craig and Sylvia" have been married 30 years. Craig had an affair that lasted three years. Sylvia found out about the affair accidentally, some months after it had ended. The affair provoked a crisis for her on several levels: She was upset about its duration, with the implication of long-term deception; she knew the "other" woman and, thus, deemed this a kind of double betrayal; the husband suffered a subsequent health crisis which delayed a timely response to the revelation of the affair; and, the husband's efforts to make changes in his current behavior were less than what she felt he "owed" her.

The therapy has lasted for almost three years and can be divided into three major therapeutic phases.

When it first became evident that Sylvia was stuck in a type of accusatory suffering, her pain and disillusionment were given priority. Then our supervisor suggested that we may have passed over the impact of the affair on her self-esteem. We returned to the very early history of the affair, its initial revelation and a review of what Sylvia needed to know about the affair to satisfy her unanswered questions. Craig was responsive to her questions, but it seemed that no amount of explanation was sufficient to calm down Sylvia's reactivity. After many couple sessions, it became clear that each effort to cover the history and meaning of the affair only intensified the gridlock. The sense of humiliation Sylvia experienced could not be reduced by any explanation or apology offered by her husband. It soon became apparent that conjoint sessions–even interspersed with individual ones–only perpetuated the gridlock.

The second phase took the form of individual sessions with both spouses. An agreement was made that the therapist would have permission to share selected information gained in both sessions with each spouse in an effort to "translate" what was being said and felt in ways that might possibly assist each partner in understanding the other. We all acknowledged that this "triangulation" technique is risky and prone to misunderstanding, but perhaps worth a try. For many subsequent sessions the therapist gave one consistent interpretation to each spouse: to Sylvia the therapist emphasized that her husband seemed sincerely contrite, but so intimidated by her easily aroused hostility that he was not sure anything he did would be sufficient. It would be more productive to try to accept his best effort as a way of encouraging more of what she wanted from him. To Craig the message was: If he avoids or walks away from Sylvia when she is angry it only convinces her that he isn't willing to deal with her intense feelings. Craig should stay with Sylvia as much as possible.

This approach worked better for Craig than his wife. She tended to see this interpretation as asking her to accept ineffectual attempts on her husband's part as enough for her to believe in him again. In a sense, the therapist was accused of encouraging her to settle for less than she felt she deserved. During these sessions, in which some of her anger was directed at the therapist, Sylvia insisted that there were many missed opportunities in which her husband did not see her obvious need for attention and respect. Craig's behaviors, she now realized, were characteristic of how he had treated her for many years. In subsequent individual sessions with Craig these "missed opportunities" were reviewed. Some, indeed, seemed to be part of his pattern of self-absorption and inattention that could well be expected to arouse his wife's anger. He seemed to understand that every missed opportunity further reinforced his wife's conviction that he really wasn't trying hard enough and that he only wanted the problems to go away. On other occasions, Craig's recollection of the events were so different from Sylvia's that it was difficult to reconcile them. Thus, two limitations of this approach became apparent: one was that discrepant interpretations of the same event could not be reconciled and the second was that when the therapist conveyed what was said and felt by one spouse to the other spouse, it could easily be heard as advocating for the absent spouse's position.

Though no great change happened in the several months of therapy in the second phase, during which Sylvia was seen much more frequently than Craig, the therapist noticed that Sylvia gradually became much less reactive during the sessions. She even seemed to develop a sense of humor about some aspects of her dilemma. She also shifted to a position that emphasized her desire to see change in how her husband treated her now and in the future. If he made significant changes, she insisted, her focus on the past infidelity would not be as acute. Thus, there was a greater willingness to work on negotiating change in painful patterns in the marriage that needed to be changed–even if the affair had never occurred. Sylvia was even open to the idea that expecting change from her husband as a condition for her to change was giving him control over the relationship–something she recognized had contributed to her low self-esteem for many years, but had only become a conscious issue in the context of the affair.

The third phase is just beginning. The plan is to resume conjoint sessions after meeting again for several individual sessions with Craig to restore some balance to the therapeutic alliance. It remains to be seen if he will be motivated to change his behavior. If he experiences Sylvia's focus as shifting from the past affair to present and future attitudes and behavior, we hope that he will seize opportunities to demonstrate his recommitment to the marriage.

WHAT WAS LEARNED

Several important insights have come from this case. The first is that accusatory suffering–as powerful as it is in its own right–cannot be separated from the relational dynamics involved. The "label" itself invites us to see it solely as the offended spouse's problem in need of being healed. What Sylvia taught us is that her suffering "at" her husband was the only strategy that seemed to keep the "heat on" for change she wanted to see come from him. Her behavior, at the same time, protected her from subsequent humiliation. The fact that it was counterproductive did not matter to her in the early stages of therapy. When she decided that she was not going to leave the marriage over the affair, a more pragmatic approach finally began to appeal to her. Sylvia reluctantly accepted her role in the stalemate without automatically assuming that she was being asked to do more than was fair to make things better. Craig had to accept that established patterns of behavior that used to be acceptable could no longer continue if he wanted to prove that he was both sorry for the affair and willing to function in a different way in the marriage.

In dealing with accusatory suffering, there is a high likelihood that therapy will degenerate into a chronic recycling of the pain of the betrayal rather than finding a path to reconciliation. When the offended spouse is given an opportunity to see how this strategy is both credible and counterproductive, there is some possibility of change. However, the offending spouse must also accept responsibility for what yet has to change in the marriage.

REFERENCES

Diagnostic criteria for 309.81 Post-traumatic Stress Disorder (1994) in *Diagnostic and statistical manual of mental disorders* (4th ed.) (pp. 427-429) Washington, DC: American Psychiatric Association.

Glass, S. (2000). *AAMFT clinical update on infidelity, 2(1),* Washington, DC: AAMFT.

Seagull, E.G., and Seagull, A.A. (1991). Healing the wound that must not heal: Psychotherapy with survivors of domestic violence. *Psychotherapy: Theory/Research/Practice/Training,* 28, 16-20.

Face It Head On:
Helping a Couple Move Through
the Painful and Pernicious Effects
of Infidelity

Adrian J. Blow

SUMMARY. This article focuses on key clinical ideas to help couples face directly the painful issues brought about by infidelity. The author discusses key relational processes related to infidelity along with desired outcomes. The emphasis is on helping couples change key relational dynamics that facilitate the healing process. Couples are encouraged to engage in the healing process head on, and not avoid or skirt around the issues. The article illustrates these desired changes by means of a case study. *[Article copies available for a fee from The Haworth Document Delivery Service: 1-800-HAWORTH. E-mail address: <docdelivery@haworthpress.com> Website: <http://www.HaworthPress.com> © 2005 by The Haworth Press, Inc. All rights reserved.]*

Adrian J. Blow, PhD, is affiliated with the Department of Counseling and Family Therapy, Saint Louis University, Saint Louis, MO.

Address correspondence to: Adrian J. Blow, PhD, Saint Louis University Department of Counseling and Family Therapy, 3750 Lindell Boulevard, Saint Louis, MO 63108 (E-mail: blowaj@slu.edu).

[Haworth co-indexing entry note]: "Face It Head On: Helping a Couple Move Through the Painful and Pernicious Effects of Infidelity." Blow, Adrian J. Co-published simultaneously in *Journal of Couple & Relationship Therapy* (The Haworth Press) Vol. 4, No. 2/3, 2005, pp. 91-102; and: *Handbook of the Clinical Treatment of Infidelity* (ed: Fred P. Piercy, Katherine M. Hertlein, and Joseph L. Wetchler) The Haworth Press, Inc., 2005, pp. 91-102. Single or multiple copies of this article are available for a fee from The Haworth Document Delivery Service [1-800-HAWORTH, 9:00 a.m. - 5:00 p.m. (EST). E-mail address: docdelivery@haworthpress.com].

Available online at http://www.haworthpress.com/web/JCRT
© 2005 by The Haworth Press, Inc. All rights reserved.
doi:10.1300/J398v04n02_09

KEYWORDS. Infidelity, relational dynamics, intimacy, relationship affirmations

INTRODUCTION

Infidelity always affects relationships. For most couples, these effects are negative, painful, and have deleterious ramifications for the relationship as a whole. Therapists who work with couples are well aware of the intense pain that infidelity generates for all parties–the victim, the offender, and the "other person." For some, these painful feelings seem to be initially intense and then dissipate over time. For others the affair wounds permanently the individual's self-concept. It also forever casts a cloud of insecurity over the relationship. To make matters worse, once an infidelity has occurred in a relationship, there is no way to erase its occurrence, and as a result, the hurt from the infidelity is always lurking somewhere in the past. Even though many couples move beyond this pain to an extent, triggers may remind them of all the old hurts when least expected. Some have argued that infidelity can serve the positive purpose of reinvigorating a lifeless relationship (Myers & Leggitt, 1972). In some cases, this might be true, but even in the cases where infidelity serves to awaken a dead or dying relationship, it leaves a residue of painful feelings.

In this article, I focus on ways couples can move beyond the pain of infidelity. This happens by allowing the event to become a part of a process that draws them closer together through empathy and understanding instead of pushing them apart through anger, insecurity, jealousy, and defensiveness. I will present some foundational points related to infidelity and then discuss fundamental relational dynamics that need to change if the couple is to "make it" in their relationship. These ideas I draw from my clinical experience with this population as well as from my reviews of the research literature on both infidelity (Blow & Hartnett, 2004a; 2004b) and couples therapy. I illustrate these points with a case study. Even though research evidence is not the basis of this article, I demonstrate the relevance of these principles in the success of one case. These ideas may not rigidly apply to every couple but their principles can certainly relate to any couple.

THE IMPACT OF INFIDELITY
ON A COMMITTED RELATIONSHIP

Infidelity always impacts a committed relationship. I suggest two fundamental points that are important for the clinician to consider in working with these couples.

Relational Dynamics of a Couple Around Infidelity Mirror Other Relational Dynamics

A common assumption is that infidelity changes the established dynamics of the couple's relationship. This might be true in some cases, but in my experience, *preexisting characteristics* of individuals in the relationship, as well as the dynamics of the relationship as a whole, predict the ways in which the couple negotiates the infidelity. For example, an insecure individual is likely to become even more insecure because of the discovery of infidelity. A defensive individual does not become less defensive as a result of an infidelity situation, and a pursue-distance relationship dynamic does not become a distance-pursue relationship dynamic. Individuals who did not like to talk about issues in the past are likely to avoid talking about the infidelity as well. Either they will want to bury the issue and move on, or they will simply avoid or be unable to talk about this difficult topic. The pursuer in the relationship will likely try to get his or her partner to talk about (and endlessly process) the occurrence of the infidelity. This may lead to increasing frustration for both parties.

Couple and family therapists strive to intervene in the process of a couple's relationship in order to bring about change. This is no different when it comes to infidelity. In working with these couples, it is important to remember that the process around the infidelity mirrors the same process in other parts of the relationship. Even though the content issues around the infidelity are painful, and intense, it is ultimately the relationship dynamics that need to be altered. This is similar to the elicitation window idea of Schnarch (1995) who relates relational dynamics to sexual dynamics in the bedroom. Frequently, individuals process the infidelity in the same way as they talk about their finances, careers, and child rearing (Blow, Morrison, Wright, Schaafsma, & Van Gundy, 2003). This idea brings to the forefront that the ultimate goal in changing relational issues is to change fundamental relational dynamics or processes of both individuals and the relationship. This has important implications for the clinician in that it is far more helpful in the long run to help a couple negotiate the process of their relational dynamics than the content issues of the infidelity. There are many content related issues when it comes to infidelity and it is possible that content details swamp the therapist, leaving pertinent process dynamics unaddressed.

Infidelity Brings Out the Most Noxious Aspects of Relationships

The research on couples and couples therapy has highlighted relationship variables that are harmful to committed relationships. John Gottman's (1999) research has stressed the toxic effects of criticism, contempt, defensiveness, and stonewalling—also known as the four horsemen. I have rarely worked with a couple dealing with infidelity in which the four horsemen were not present in some way. Infidelity seems to make these harmful processes worse, and in some cases, it gives the individuals a license to introduce them into their relationship. For example, the victim of infidelity might believe that his or her partner deserves to suffer an equal amount of pain and barrage the partner with a constant assault of criticism and contempt. This often serves no more purpose than to heighten the degree of defensiveness and stonewalling in the person who is attacked.

Susan Johnson, one of the developers of emotionally focused couples therapy is a strong advocate of the role of emotional processes in relationships based on attachment perspectives (Johnson, 1996; see Susan Johnson's paper elsewhere in this volume). She believes that it is a change in the emotional processes of a relationship that lead to changes in relational dynamics. Further, she achieves this by moving couples away from "hard feelings" such as anger, frustration, and hatred towards "softer feelings" that are more palatable and connecting like sadness, hurt, and fear. She further talks about attachment injuries in relationships and the ways in which couples therapy can serve to heal some of these injuries through changing the way people relate. Conversely, ineffective relating may deepen these attachment injuries (Johnson, Makinen, & Millikin, 2001).

Few other issues are as emotionally charged as infidelity. Further, when it comes to basic attachment needs, infidelity injures fundamental qualities (not dynamics) of a relationship, and is incredibly threatening to both the survival needs of an individual as well as of a relationship. As a result, individuals hurt by infidelity often resort to survival tactics, revenge, and raw emotions, characterized by anger and hostility, along with criticism, contempt, and defensiveness. All therapists who have worked with infidelity are familiar with the emotional roller coaster

(Olson, Russell, Higgins-Kessler, & Miller, 2002) that comes with the infidelity territory. Infidelity invokes some of the scariest emotions in an individual. Both murder and suicide have occurred because of infidelity, and everything else in between. Even though these are strong emotions and it is always a trying time, it can also be an opportunity for deep relational healing to occur both in the lives of the individuals and in the relationship as a whole.

DESIRED PROCESS OUTCOME

Although these desired process outcomes (like sharing hurt versus anger) are global in nature, they are easily adapted to specific therapist styles and couple issues. Even though a discussion of content issues related to infidelity is always necessary, and different clinicians have different ideas on how much content needs to be discussed (i.e., every sordid detail of the infidelity versus a minimal discussion of details), it is ultimately the relating process of the couple that needs to change for healing to occur.

Infidelity Issues Are Best Dealt With Head On

Many individuals are quite good at avoiding difficult issues in their relationships. They often do this by simply not talking about or talking around the subject. Talking about the issues related to the infidelity is always intense, emotional, and painful. However, with time, these intensities seem to diminish allowing a more open process to result (Glass & Wright, 1997). Couples who avoid talking about the painful issues, never seem to arrive at the open process that allows for higher levels of relational intimacy to occur. Couples need to face directly the issues related to infidelity if the relationship is to stand any chance of intimacy, even though these are intense issues. Some couples are not willing to face these issues head on, and there are many couples who would rather not talk about them again. Even though these couples can and do have satisfactory relationships, for the most part, they cannot avoid these issues if they desire deeper levels of intimacy. Further, the couple needs to know that the healing from infidelity is not overnight. A general rule is that it takes time, and in some cases, years, to get back on track again. However, great levels of intimacy can arise out of the process of working through the painful issues.

Infidelity Is a Unique Relational Event Separate from Other Relational Issues

One of the strategies that couples can use to deal with infidelity is to treat it as a unique relational event. By this, I mean that in every relationship there are issues separate from the infidelity that may be gridlocked, perpetual, and sometimes painful (Gottman, 1999). These include subjects like finances, child-rearing, career choices, in-laws, and the like. When infidelity occurs, it is common for the offending party to lose power and status in these other important relationship areas. While in the short term this may work, it is not an ideal long-term arrangement. This is why I believe that treating the infidelity as a unique relational event separate from these other issues is important. For example, as will be discussed next, the offending party should always take an apologetic stance around the infidelity injury. However, this does not mean that the offending party is automatically one down in all other aspects of the relationship, but rather that these are separate relational issues. Keeping the infidelity as a unique relational event that is separate from other relational negotiations/issues prevents new issues emerging in the relationship in the long run. It also prevents the victim of infidelity taking advantage of the situation and making unilateral decisions that affect the entire family. In addition, it allows the offending party to engage around the infidelity in an open and honest way without feeling that he or she is losing all status in the relationship.

Actions Required of the Offending Party

There are some actions that the offending party can take to help the relationship heal if he or she is committed to making the relationship work. Ideally, this is not a simple linear, black or white process.

A Life-Long Apologetic Stance Around the Infidelity

The offending party often asks, "How many times must I say I am sorry?" My answer is, "As many times as is necessary." It is important that this apologetic stance is specifically focused on the infidelity and that other relational transgressions are kept separate. It is also important that the offending party know that a defensive stance around the infidelity is never helpful, that the partner's feelings are real and legitimate, and that what they did lead to deep relational and individual hurts. The offending party cannot apologize too many times in regard to the infidelity, and he or she may indeed need to apologize periodically for the remainder of the relationship. Common reactions of the offending party are "Do you mean I am going to live with this for the rest of my life?" The easy answer is "Yes." The more difficult answer is explaining why this is true. It is true in essence because the ongoing apologetic stance represents a process shift in the relational dynamics around a painful issue. It also serves to avoid any polarizations from occurring around the infidelity. Finally, it serves to provide a secure base for the victim of infidelity in that he or she will always feel safe to bring up the issue knowing that it will lead to reassurance of some sort and not frustration or defensiveness. The victim of infidelity may completely avoid bringing up the subject of the infidelity if he or she believes that talking about fears and hurts will bring up defensiveness and frustration.

Soft feelings that are genuine best characterize the apologetic stance. This is right in line with the ideas of Susan Johnson (1996), who moves couples into a soft place where they can hear each other and communicate with genuine feelings. It is common for the offending party to communicate from a place of shame, guilt, or defensiveness. These are not helpful to the overall relational process. An example of a soft interaction would be, "I hurt you, and I was wrong. I am unhappy with myself that I allowed this to happen. I understand that you are hurt. I know that what I did was incredibly painful, wrong, and hurtful to you and our relationship, and I am truly sorry."

The apologetic stance is best if accompanied by validation and understanding. Validation and understanding are particularly important in the healing process. This process involves letting the victim of infidelity know that his or her feelings are real and understandable and that he or she has every right to feel the way that he or she does. An example of validation and healing would be, "I understand that you are feeling really anxious right now thinking about what I did to you. It makes sense to me that you would feel this way." It is important to remember that feelings are feelings and they are best solved through validation–not frustration or belittlement.

The apologetic stance is best if accompanied by a relationship affirmation addressing security needs. It is important that the offending party is aware that what he or she did constituted a major attachment threat to the relationship (Johnson, Makinen, & Millikin, 2001). The feelings of insecurity and jealousy are quite likely to be present in the hurt party. A way in which the offending party can address these security needs is to say, "Even though I have hurt you in the past, I want to reassure you that I love you and that you are the one whom I choose to be with the remainder of my life."

The Actions Required of the Victim of Infidelity

Even though the non-offending party did nothing wrong, he or she has a key role to play in helping the couple heal. What follows are some shifts that the non-offending party can make.

A Move Away from Criticism and Contemptuous Interactions to a Focus on Hurts, Losses, and Fears

This shift especially relates to concerns and insecurities that the victim has related to the infidelity. It is understandable that for a time, the victim of infidelity will express these concerns in angry ways, but at some point, the non-offending partner needs to realize that concerns about the infidelity expressed in critical, contemptuous, or with hard emotions need to end if healing is to occur. So ideally, the non-offending partner needs to move to a place where he or she is able to talk about fears, hurts, and insecurities without lashing out in unhelpful ways.

Realistic Forgiveness Stance Around Infidelity

At some point in the process, the couple will move into a place where they are ready to move ahead in the relationship through a forgiveness process. It is essential that there is a realistic forgiveness stance around infidelity. It is important in the forgiveness process to remember that the hurt of the infidelity will always be present to an extent. Also, it is important to remember that the infidelity has forever changed the relationship. It is also helpful for the non-offending party to know that the offending party will never feel the same amount of pain that he or she does and that to wish hurt on their partner only hurts more in the long run. The infidelity injury realistically is not something that the offending party needs to be reminded of every second of every day. At some point, the intensity needs to diminish if true forgiveness is to occur.

Relationship Affirmations Addressing Security Needs

Similar to the offending partner, it is helpful that the victim of infidelity is able to get to a point where he or she can address the security needs of the offending spouse. In many cases, the act of infidelity makes the offending spouse feel that the relationship is over and he or she can feel very insecure. Both partners need to be willing to reassure each other about their love for each other, their choice to be with each other, and the security of their relationship. An example of what the victim of infidelity can say is, "What you did really hurt me to my core. However, I have realized that you are the one I love and that I wish to spend the rest of my life with. I realize that you could hurt me all over again, and if that happened, I would leave you. However, I am willing to give you and our relationship a second chance."

A Realistic Realization About the Ability to Control the Occurrence of Future Infidelities

It is helpful for the victim of infidelity to realize that there is nothing that he or she can do to prevent the infidelity from reoccurring should the partner wish to cheat again. This belief helps the individual know that feeling insecure and vulnerable as a result of the infidelity leads to the desire to control every action of one's partner. It makes more sense for the offended party to develop a clear plan of action as to what he or she would do should the infidelity reoccur.

What if the Victim of Infidelity Is Stuck and Unable to Move Forward?

There are times when the victim of infidelity is stuck and is just not able to move beyond the pain of what has happened. Four questions are helpful to ask and explore in investigating the impasse of the individual. Is the offending party genuine in his or her soft stance? Is the offending party dismissive of the feelings of his or her partner in an effort to put it all in the past? Is the infidelity really over? Are their other issues in the past (such as previous infidelities in other relationships or current relationship, or parental infidelities) that contribute to impasses around infidelity?

CASE STUDY ILLUSTRATION

The Case

Michael and Madison, a heterosexual couple, had been married for 28 years. They had three children, all at college. They presented in therapy because Michael had discovered a suspicious email on his wife's laptop when he had been looking for a family recipe. He had confronted her about the email and she confessed that she had been having an affair with another woman for a long time. When Michael confronted her about how long, she admitted that it had been for at least 20 years but she was unsure as to exactly when it began. Michael was devastated. He had always been the pursuer in the relationship. He had wanted them to spend more time together as a couple over the years and had been particularly unhappy with their sexual relationship. In the first ten years of the marriage, he had continually "pestered" Madison for more sex, but she had continually rebuffed him. At a point, Michael stopped asking and had resorted to masturbation approximately three times weekly to take care of his sexual frustrations. He had thought of Madison as having little to no sexual interest. Now, her infidelity had brought up years of marital frustration. He began to reinterpret everything that they had done together over the years as tainted and wasted. He felt like he had been living a lie. It also served to bring up two earlier relationships prior to his marriage in which his girlfriends had cheated on him. Further, his father had regularly cheated on his mother and when he was a child, Michael had often found himself caught up in the middle of his parents' arguments over his father's infidelity. As a result of the discovery of the infidelity, Madison was scared and vulnerable. For years, she felt that she had been unable to talk to Michael about their issues. Her preferred style of relating was to avoid issues, bottling up her emotions, and she ended up stonewalling him. She had long felt frustrated in her sexual relationship with Michael. She found him to be rough and uncaring. She had met her lover at work (her lover was also married) and the relationship had developed into a sexual encounter filled with tenderness and passion. However, it had limited emotional connection, and neither had ever planned to leave their marriages to be with each other. She reported that she still loved Michael very much, he was her best friend, they had much in common, and that she was willing to end the infidelity to save the marriage.

The Therapy Process

In this case, several significant issues occurred that helped the couple to reengage with each other. In the first place, after Michael first found out abut the infidelity he was hurt and lashed out repeatedly at Madison. He did not hold back on his verbal assaults and Madison was regularly in tears. However, at this point Michael also decided that this was a relationship that he at least wanted to try to save and he asked Madison if she would go to marital therapy. He had asked her ten years earlier if she would go to therapy to talk about their sex life at which time she had refused, stating that therapy was for crazy people and that it would bring great shame to her family. However, this time Madison agreed to go. This was a significant step for Michael and he viewed it as a sign of her intent to try. At this point, I received the phone call and we set up a time to meet.

Therapy was difficult for Madison. Her preferred style of relating had always been from a defensive place, and she found therapy intense and uncomfortable. However, in spite of this, she attended faithfully and was, for the most, always engaged in the process. As painful as it was for both parties to talk about the issues, I urged them to stay engaged around their issues and not to "bail out" as they had in the past. They attended therapy for 90 minutes each week. They also set aside three hours each Saturday afternoon to talk about what had happened. This was a painful process, and there were always tears from both parties. Michael complained that he again found himself in a pursuer role and felt as if he had to dig things out of Madison. He wanted her to talk openly about the details of what had occurred even though this was not comfortable for her to do. I coached Madison on how to deal with Michael's feelings. When he was feeling hurt and insecure, she would look him in the eyes and say, "Michael, I am so sorry for what I did to you. It was wrong and I take responsibility for my actions. I want to make things right with you. I know what I did will always be a part of our relationship but I realize that I love you very much and want to spend the rest of my life with you." When Madison said this, it always calmed Michael down and they found themselves able to connect at this point in the process. When it came to the subject of the infidelity, Madison was able to take an apologetic stance from a sincere place. When she talked, I sensed that she was genuine. Over time, both individuals began to feel increasingly secure in their relationship. They also began to experience a connecting sex life for the first time.

Two years after the discovery of the infidelity, Michael continued to experience bouts of emotion related to what had happened, especially around certain triggers. When Michael would spiral down, Madison was unable to calm him down, and he was unable to calm himself down. When this happened, Michael began some individual work in the presence of Madison in which he was able to revisit his painful triangulation as a child and rejections from his earlier partners. It was only then that he was able to move out of his stuck place. After he had dealt with these issues, he still had times of insecurity but the reassurance of Madison helped him get through these times. At this writing, the couple reports that things are still going very well in their relationship and that even though it all still hurts, they are closer and more content with each other than before.

REFERENCES

Blow, A. J., & Hartnett, K. (under review). Infidelity in committed relationships I: A methodological review. Submitted to *Journal of Marital & Family Therapy*.

Blow, A. J., & Hartnett, K. (under review). Infidelity in long-term committed relationships II: A substantive review. Submitted to *Journal of Marital & Family Therapy*.

Blow, A. J., Morrison, N. C., Wright, K. A., Schaafsma, M. C., & Van Gundy, A. E. (2003). *Progress Research and Change Processes in Couples Therapy*. Presentation at the American Association for Marital and Family Therapy Conference.

Glass, S. P., & Wright, T. L. (1997). Reconstructing marriages after the trauma of infidelity. In W. K. Halford & H. J. Markman (Eds.), *Clinical handbook of marriage and couples interventions* (pp. 471-507). New York: Wiley.

Gottman, J. M. (1999). *The marriage clinic: A scientifically based marital therapy*. NY: Norton.

Johnson, S. M. (1996). *The practice of emotionally focused marital therapy: Creating connection*. New York: Brunner/Mazel.

Johnson, S. M., Makinen, J. A., & Millikin, J. W. (2001). Attachment injuries in couple relationships: A new perspective on impasses in couples therapy. *Journal of Marital & Family Therapy, 27,* 145-156.

Myers, L., & Leggitt, H. (1972). A new kind of adultery. *Sexual Behavior, 2,* 52-62.

Olson, M. M., Russell, C. S., Higgins-Kessler, M., & Miller, R. B. (2002). Emotional processes following disclosure of an extramarital infidelity. *Journal of Marital & Family Therapy, 28(4),* 423-434.

Schnarch, D. (1995). *Passionate marriage: Love, sex, and intimacy in emotionally committed relationships*. New York: Norton.

Taking the Good with the Bad:
Applying Klein's Work
to Further Our Understandings
of Cyber-Cheating

Monica T. Whitty
Adrian N. Carr

SUMMARY. Although there is a paucity of research available on cyber-cheating and its effects on the offline couple, the current research available suggests that Internet relationships and online erotic interac-

Dr. Monica T. Whitty is Lecturer, School of Psychology, Queen's University Belfast, Northern Ireland, UK.

Dr. Adrian N. Carr is Associate Professor, School of Applied Social and Human Sciences, University of Western Sydney, Australia.

Address correspondence to: Dr. Monica Whitty, Queen's University Belfast, School of Psychology, David Keir Building, Northern Ireland, BT7 1NN (E-mail: m.whitty@qub.ac.uk).

[Haworth co-indexing entry note]: "Taking the Good with the Bad: Applying Klein's Work to Further Our Understandings of Cyber-Cheating." Whitty, Monica T., and Adrian N. Carr. Co-published simultaneously in *Journal of Couple & Relationship Therapy* (The Haworth Press) Vol. 4, No. 2/3, 2005, pp. 103-115; and: *Handbook of the Clinical Treatment of Infidelity* (ed: Fred P. Piercy, Katherine M. Hertlein, and Joseph L. Wetchler) The Haworth Press, Inc., 2005, pp. 103-115. Single or multiple copies of this article are available for a fee from The Haworth Document Delivery Service [1-800-HAWORTH, 9:00 a.m. - 5:00 p.m. (EST). E-mail address: docdelivery@haworthpress.com].

tions can have a 'real' impact on couples. This paper builds on the current research by exploring theoretical explanations for how individuals might rationalize their online affairs. Drawing from Klein's object-relations theory we suggest that while on one level individuals might perceive their online interactions to be 'unreal' and hence not 'breaking the rules' in respect to the offline relationship, on another level energy is being taken away from the relationship and given to another, which is indeed 'breaking the rules.' *[Article copies available for a fee from The Haworth Document Delivery Service: 1-800-HAWORTH. E-mail address: <docdelivery@haworthpress.com> Website: <http://www.HaworthPress.com> © 2005 by The Haworth Press, Inc. All rights reserved.]*

KEYWORDS. Cyber-cheating, Internet infidelity, Klein, splitting, object-relations, Winnicott

Cyber-cheating is still a relatively under-researched and under-theorised topic in the social sciences. Atwood (2002) asserts that "healthcare professionals are often unfamiliar with the dynamics associated with the relatively new concept of cyber-affairs and the electronic process of 'virtual cheating' and thus often do not consider the behaviour as infidelity" (p. 37). Given this claim, it would seem that there is an urgent need to consider whether online interactions and erotic activities online are considered to be real acts of betrayal by individuals and their offline partners, and if this behaviour needs to be considered more seriously by healthcare professionals (e.g., relationship counsellors). The research, to date, suggests that cyber-affairs can have a real and possibly serious impact on the offline relationship. Whitty (2003a), for instance, found that individuals do perceive that some interactions that occur online can be considered as acts of betrayal. The study identified three main components of infidelity: *sexual*, *emotional*, and *porn*. Moreover, it was found that some acts, such as sexual acts pose a greater threat than other acts, such as viewing pornography.

In this paper, we would like to extend on current work in the field by considering theoretically the processes that might take place when people do have cyber-affairs. While we do not subscribe to the view that all online relationships and erotic acts ought to be considered acts of infidelity to all people, we are limiting this paper to considerations of the *psychological processes* that might take place when these are considered to be acts of betrayal. We firstly consider here, drawing from

Winnicott's (1971/1997) work on potential space, how cyberspace might be seen as an attractive place to play at love and that in many instances this can be therapeutic for individuals. We then turn to considerations raised by theorists, such as Civin (2000), that cyberspace can also be debilitating. We examine how online infidelities might be perceived by some to be 'unreal' acts and focus on justifications and excuses perpetrators might use to explain away these encounters. The taken-for-granted rules of a relationship are also focused on here. Drawing from the foundational object-relations work of Melanie Klein (1986), in relation to the process of *splitting*, we argue that people are more easily able to justify their online affairs when compared to their offline affairs. To illustrate our argument we provide examples, from a recent study, where individuals were asked to respond to a hypothetical scenario on cyber-cheating (Whitty, 2003c). It is noteworthy that while we would also argue that cyberspace is not limited to Internet interactions, we have restricted this paper to considerations of Internet affairs. We are of the view that attempting to understand, in greater detail, the psychological processes that take place when individuals cyber-cheat may lead to improved treatments for Internet infidelity. The paper goes some way in contributing to raising awareness of some of the more serious consequences of cyber-affairs.

Playing at Love: Object-Relations

Previously we have argued, when read through the optic of Winnicott's (1971/1997) object-relations theory, that cyberspace has potential therapeutic benefits to offer. We have suggested that cyberspace is a safe and imaginative place to play at flirting and love (Whitty, 2003b; Whitty & Carr, 2003).

Winnicott was very interested in what he called the *potential space*–a space between the mother and the infant. He contrasted this "potential space (a) with the inner world (which is related to the psychosomatic partnership) and (b) with actual, or external reality" (Winnicott, 1971/1997, p. 41). Winnicott understood 'potential spaces' to be an area of intermediate experiencing that is between inner and outer worlds, "between the subjective object and the object objectively perceived" (Winnicott, 1971/1997, p. 100). Winnicott (1971/1997) argued that the potential space is:

> the hypothetical area that exists (but cannot exist) between the baby and the object (mother of part of mother) during the phase of

> the repudiation of the object as not-me, that is, at the end of being merged in with the object. (p. 107)

Winnicott noticed, for example, how an infant would suck and hug a doll or blanket. He suggested that the doll or blanket did not represent a doll or blanket as such, but is rather *an as-if object*. The infant makes use of the illusion that although this is not the breast, treating it as such will allow an appreciation of what is "me" and what is "not-me" (Winnicott, 1971/1997, p. 41). Although referred to as a transitional object, "it is not the object, of course that is transitional" (Winnicott, 1971/1997, p. 14). The object is the initial manifestation of a different positioning of the infant in the world. The doll or blanket, thus, connects to subjective experience, but is in the objective world.

While the notions of transitional objects and potential space are raised within a context of an infant, Winnicott (1971/1997) insists, however, they are not simply confined to the infant's experience, but is something that "throughout life is retained in the intense experiencing that belongs to the arts and to religion and to imaginative living, and to creative scientific work" (p. 24). We come to rely upon our own resources to experience culture to expand our understanding of the world. In his expanded views on mental health and creativity, Winnicott argues that a person who lives in a realm of subjective omnipotence, with no bridge to objective reality, is self-absorbed and autistic. A person who lived only in the realm of objective reality, with no roots in subjective omnipotence, was viewed by Winnicott as superficially adjusted, but lacking passion and originality. This realm provides relief "from the strain of relating inner and outer reality . . . that no human is free from" (Winnicott, 1971/1997, p. 24). The tension and strain between inner and outer worlds is not eliminated, but is bound in this space. Culture and cultural activity, in this context, is an expression of the "inter-play between separateness and union" (Winnicott, 1971/1997, p. 24).

The potential space is not pure fantasy, nor is it pure reality. "In the absence of potential space, there is only fantasy; within potential space imagination can develop" (Ogden, 1985, p. 133). Winnicott believed that given a 'good enough' environment the interplay of the inner world and external reality promotes the development of self and facilitates growth. It is a space where we can develop psychologically, to integrate love and hate and to create, destroy, and re-create ourselves (see Winnicott, 1971/1997, p. 41).

In line with Winnicott's object-relations theory, we have suggested that cyberspace is a potential space (Whitty, 2003b; Whitty & Carr,

2003). Cyberspace, like Winnicott's potential space is perhaps a space somewhere outside the individual, but is still not the external world. The participants and their transitional objects: the computers, monitors, keyboards, mice, software, modems, text, cables, telephone lines, and so forth; all occupy this potential space–a space between the 'real individuals' and the 'fantasy individuals.'

We have argued that flirting is a type of play that can occur in this potential space–cyberspace. Cyber-flirting, although akin in some ways with offline flirting, is characterised here as a *unique activity* that is a form of play. Of course it can be argued, with justification, that offline flirting is also a form of play. That said, cyberspace seems to offer more opportunities for the type of play that Winnicott described. Similarly, cyberspace offers opportunities for this play to be transformational. We have expressed this view given that offline flirting requires that another be physically present. In face-to-face interactions rejection is more possible and probably more damaging to one's self concept. Cyberspace, in contrast, gives to many the appearance of a safer environment; a safer space to play and experiment at flirting. Moreover, rejection is less likely to cause distress when you can disconnect at any time, and the chances are remarkably decreased as to the likelihood of ever having a chance meeting with one's cyber-playmate.

A Darker Side of the Internet

While contending that cyberspace can be potentially a therapeutic place to play at love we have also acknowledged that cyberspace also has its dark side (Whitty & Carr, 2003). We would also not dismiss the notion that engaging in intimate relationships or erotic acts online might even have a positive effect (at least for the person engaging in these activities). However, in the context of this paper, like Civin (2000), we would like to propose that "Just as cyberspace may potentiate, it may also thwart and debilitate" (p. 40).

Civin (2000) proposes that cyberspace is not as transitional and facilitative as it was first considered by academics. Perhaps this is because of the changing nature of this space, or possibly this is because the darker aspects of cyberspace were not taken into account by early researchers. Civin (2000) has brought to our attention that ". . . no object or process, the cyber system included is essentially transitional" (p. 39). Continuing this line of argument, he reminds the reader that Winnicott was not suggesting that all teddy bears and blankets are essentially transitional! Likewise, not all cyber systems will act as transitional objects! He adds that, in stark contrast, cyber systems are potentially invasive, so much so that they can foster persecutory anxiety. Civin states, that for some, "the computer system seems a far cry (in all meanings) from the teddy bear or favorite blanket, and the breach between the cyber system and the transitional or potential looms unnegotiably vast" (2000, p. 51).

Civin (2000) presents the reader with case studies to illustrate how the cyber system can foster persecutory anxiety. For example, in his presentation of the online experiences of a person he calls Jeannette, Civin demonstrates how she was eventually forced off the net after she angered someone for sharing software he had sent to her. This rage changed to jealousy and Jeannette found she was being e-mailed more frequently than she could cope with and, in addition, feared her husband would eventually discover her online relationships. Other examples of deleterious effects of cyberspace might include harassment, cyberstalking, and addiction. This paper, however, examines the problems that arise when individuals engage in cyber-affairs.

Melanie Klein: 'Good' and 'Bad' Objects

We would like to suggest here, that while the motivations for an online affair might be similar to why individuals seek affairs offline (e.g., problems encountered in the relationships, personality factors) the appeal and the way the online relationship is perceived can be potentially different. We would argue that online affairs may appear to be in some ways more seductive than offline affairs.

To explain this we would like to draw from Melanie Klein's work on splitting. Splitting, she believed, was one of the most primitive or basic defence mechanisms against anxiety. According to Klein (1986), the ego prevents the 'bad' part of the object from contaminating the 'good' part of the object by splitting it off and disowning a part of itself. An infant in its relationship with the mother's breast conceives it as both a good and bad object. The breast gratifies and frustrates and the infant will simultaneously project both love and hate on to it. On the one hand the infant idealises this 'good' object, but on the other hand, the 'bad' object is seen as terrifying, frustrating and a persecutor threatening to destroy both the infant and the 'good' object (Carr, 1997). The infant projects love and idealises the good object but goes beyond mere projection in trying to induce in the mother feelings toward the bad object for which she must take responsibility (that is, a process of projective identification). This stage of development Klein termed the *paranoid-*

schizoid position. The infant may, as another defence mechanism for this less developed ego, seek to deny the reality of the persecutory object. While in the normal development we pass through this phase, this primitive defence against anxiety is a regressive reaction that, in a sense of always being available to us, is never transcended. The 'good' objects in the developed super-ego come to represent the fantasized ego-ideal and thus "the possibility of a return to narcissism" (Schwartz, 1990, p. 18).

In line with Klein's object-relations theory it might be useful to understand the individual with whom one is having an online affair to be the 'good object.' Given that the interactions that take place in cyberspace can be seen as separate to the outside world it is potentially easier to split an online affair off from the rest of the individual's world. As we will elaborate on further in this paper, the online relationship can potentially cater to an unfettered, impotent fantasy that is difficult to measure up to in reality. Hence, the online affair can potentially lead to a narcissistic withdrawal.

Relationship Scripts

Engaging in extra-dyadic relationships is considered by most individuals, at least in Western countries, to be an act of betrayal. It is generally taken-for-granted by heterosexual couples that engaging in an intimate relationship with someone other than one's partner, especially in respect to sexual activities, is unacceptable and a breach of the rules of the relationship. Research has found that sexual infidelity is one of the most common causes of marital break-ups (e.g., Betzig, 1989; Pittman & Wagers, 1995). In fact, Pittman and Wagers (1995) found that, in their clinical experience, more than 90% of divorces were attributed to sexual infidelity.

While heterosexuals might have scripts available to them as to what are acceptable face-to-face interactions with the opposite sex while still maintaining a romantic relationship, given the nature and the newness of the Internet, the rules are yet to be clearly established as to what are acceptable online encounters. Although it has been found that individuals hold similar attitudes towards online and offline infidelities (Whitty, 2003a), more recent work has found that when presented with a hypothetical scenario of a partner potentially cheating online, that not all participants were convinced that this was 'real' betrayal (Whitty, 2003c). In the study referred to here, participants were given one of two versions of a story-completion task based on a task devised about traditional offline infidelity by Kitzinger and Powell (1995). They were presented with one of the versions presented below:

> *Version A:* Mark and Jennifer have been going out for over a year. Then Mark realizes that Jennifer has developed a relationship with someone else over the Internet. . .
> *Version B:* Jennifer and Mark have been going out for over a year. Then Jennifer realizes that Mark has developed a relationship with someone else over the Internet. . .

While Kitzinger and Powell (1995) found that 90% of their sample interpreted their cue story, which was developed in respect to offline infidelity, to be an act of sexual involvement, this was not the case in this particular study. While all of the participants understood this to be a dilemma about infidelity, some were divided as to whether the betrayer believed they were committing an act of infidelity, while others wrote that the partner was not certain that they had been betrayed. Moreover, unlike Kitzinger and Powell's study, when participants interpreted the cue story as a story about sexual involvement, this was not necessarily about a sexual relationship, but in many cases was exclusively an emotional involvement.

Although the majority of the participants (86%) wrote in their stories that the aggrieved felt that they had been betrayed, and 51% wrote that the betrayer believed that they had been unfaithful, a number of participants were uncertain that this was a scenario about infidelity. Explanations given as to why the scenario should not be considered as infidelity were that:

- the interaction was 'just a friendship';
- the interaction was merely flirtation or fun;
- the relationship was with an object (computer) in virtual space, rather than with a real human being;
- the interaction was with two people who had never met and did not ever intend to meet; and,
- it could not be infidelity as there was no physical sex taking place.

Given that the results from this study present somewhat different results to the Kitzinger and Powell's study on offline infidelity, this suggests that there is something different about the relationships we form online. This can be partly attributed to some people's beliefs that these relationships are not completely real. As illustrated in the following quote elicited from the study mentioned above:

> *Mark at first brushes it off thinking that it's "only the Internet, no harm in having fun."* (12MM)

Fitness (2001) has pointed out that the key to defining betrayal lies in "relationship knowledge structures"; for example, individuals' theories, beliefs, and expectations about how relationships should normally work and how their own relationships should work. Given that the types of interactions that take place online are somewhat different and perhaps in some ways feel less real than offline relationships, it might be that virtual sex and developing close emotional bonds with someone online might be perceived by some as not breaking the rules of the offline relationship. However, in saying this, we would like to suggest that acts of infidelity are not necessarily limited to sexual acts, such as sexual intercourse, kissing and so forth. Rather, part of the expectations of a relationship can be both *'mental exclusivity'* as well as *'sexual exclusivity'* (Yarab, Sensibaugh, & Allgeier, 1998). As Fitness (2001) also contends:

> Essentially, betrayal means that one party in a relationship acts in a way that favours his or her own interests at the expense of the other party's interests. In one sense, this behaviour implies that the betrayer regards his or her needs as more important than the needs of the partner or the relationship. In a deeper sense, however, betrayal sends an ominous signal about how little the betrayer cares about, or values his or her relationship with, the betrayed partner. (p. 73)

Hence, if acts of betrayal are not limited to 'real' sexual acts then it is quite plausible to consider various types of online relating to be construed as acts of infidelity by the offline couple.

This notion that online acts can be considered as acts of betrayal is nicely summarised in the following extract:

"It is cheating." She said rather calmly.
"No I'm not cheating. It's not like I'm bonking her anyway. You're the one I'm with and like I said I have <u>NO</u> intentions of meeting her." He hopped into bed.
"It's 'emotional' cheating." She said getting annoyed.

"How so?" He asked, amusement showing in his eyes.
"Cheating isn't necessarily physical. That's one side of it . . ." He
pulled the sheets over him and rolled over.
"Well. . . I know you have not met her yet that's why, but I'm still a little
annoyed, Mark." She sat on the edge of the bed.
"Don't be mad. You're the one I love. So how is it emotional cheating?"
He sat up.
"You're keeping stuff from me. Relationships are about trust! How can
I trust you if you keep stuff from me about the 'Internet' girl'?" (51FM)

Online Relationships: Fantasy or Reality?

If we are to take on the argument that cyberspace can be perceived in
a similar way to Winnicott's understanding of potential space (see
Whitty, 2003b; Whitty & Carr, 2003) then while potential space does
offer greater opportunities to flirt and play at love, these relationships
are not complete fantasy. We would like to suggest here that given the
lack of scripts currently available as to what is acceptable behaviour online and given the nature of cyberspace, some individuals might find it
easier to justify or rationalize engaging in an online affair. On one level
the relationship or sexual encounter can be seen as fantasy and not real.
However, at another level, the relationship or sexual encounter can be
understood as hurting the offline relationship. Therefore, in line with
Melanie Klein's work, we would like to propose that splitting is easier
to do in respect to online infidelity than offline infidelity.

Fitness (2001) contends that there are four main ways that individuals account for their betrayal: (a) conceding that an offence has been
committed accompanied by remorse and possibly an attempt to re-establish the relationship; (b) an admittance of the offence together with
excuses of extenuating circumstances, such as alcohol, stress, and illness; (c) in a more defensive account where the offence is admitted,
however, the offender minimizes its wrongness or seriousness; and,
(d) denials of having committed any offence or refusals to take any responsibility for it.

While the stories in Whitty's study (2003c) demonstrated examples
of each of these accounts, a unique finding that emerged was that when
excuses were made, they were typically along the lines of the relationship not being real. However, when confronted with this excuse the ag-
grieved would still see that an act of betrayal had occurred and as a

consequence trust had been broken. This is exemplified in the following extracts:

> *When she confronts him about it one night over dinner, he denies ev-erything saying that they were just friends. And that she should not take it so seriously and worry about it because it was not a real relationship, but a net relationship. That net relationships mean nothing because ev-eryone lives in virtual reality. Jennifer accepts his theory, but decides to leave him in the end, her departing words are, "I'm sorry Mark, but I can't be with someone who wants to live in virtual reality with some-one, and in reality with me."* (6FM)

> *She tried to explain that he was just a faithful companion and the only feelings he had were not real as this man was just words on a screen, but he couldn't understand the relationship and why she would need to tell others of their private lives.* (55FJ)

Interestingly, the second extract raises another expectation of an offline re-lationship; that there are some aspects of the offline relationship that ought to remain private and not shared with others. Part of the objection the ag-grieved seems to have here is that the perpetrator has inverted priorities.

It has been argued that offline infidelity occurs because there are prob-lems in the relationship, or because of certain personality characteristics (see Fitness, 2001). Buss and Shackelford (1997) have identified some key reasons why people betray their partners, including: complaints that one's partner sexualizes others; exhibits high levels of jealousy and possessive-ness; is condescending; sexual withholding; and, abuses alcohol. Of greater interest to this paper is that Buss and Shackelford found a strong link be-tween narcissism and susceptibility to infidelity. These are perhaps the same reasons why individuals are motivated to initiate online affairs. However, drawing from Klein's theory, we would like to suggest that these relationships are perhaps easier to maintain than an offline affair. We contend that the online relationship can become idealized through the process of splitting, while simultaneously, denying the 'bad' aspects of the person they are having the affair with and at the same time the bad as-pects in themselves. It is possibly easier to idealise an individual online (the 'good' object) when you can more easily filter out the potential nega-tive aspects of the relationship (the 'bad' object). The relationship can be turned on or off at one's leisure and the communication content, to some extent, can be more easily controlled. Moreover, the Internet does pro-vide an environment where it is easier to construct a more positive view of the self and avoid presenting the negative aspects of the self. In contrast, it is not so easy to indulge in one's fantasies of perfection in an offline affair as one has to still deal with the 'real' person.

The work of Christopher Bollas is also useful to consider here. Bollas (1987) described how the search for the idealised lover can be a quest to compensate for a deficiency in the ego. As he states:

> Some forms of erotomania may be efforts to establish the other as the transformational object. The search for the perfect crime or the perfect woman is not only a quest for an idealized object. It also constitutes some recognition in the subject of a deficiency in ego experience. The search, even though it serves to split the bad experience from the subject's cognitive knowledge, is nonetheless a semiological act that signifies the person's search for a particular object relation that is associated with ego transformation and repair of the 'basic fault.' (Bollas, 1987, p. 18)

In line with Bollas's thinking, cyberspace provides more radical opportunities to find that perfect object, the object that resonates with the good aspects of oneself and that allows one to disregard the 'bad' objects that perhaps the offline lover is more inclined to bring to one's attention. Also, given the potential anonymous nature of the Internet, one is less likely to be caught out engaging in online infidelities. Hence, as argued earlier, cyberspace does in many ways provide one with *a safer place* to play at love. Moreover, as Cooper (1998) contends, three factors that make the Internet such a powerful medium for online sexual activities, include 'access,' 'affordability,' and 'anonymity.' Taken together these aspects suggests that cyberspace is not only a different place for infidelities to be acted out but possibly a more attractive space to engage in such activities–in spite of that absence of 'real' physical sex.

In conclusion, we believe that despite the lack of real bodies in cyberspace, online affairs can have a real impact on the offline relationship. We have raised the notion here that, given the nature of cyberspace, individuals might be more easily able to rationalize their online betrayals, however, this does not necessarily make the betrayal any less severe. Moreover, online relationships have a certain seductive appeal which in some ways could be potentially more damaging to an offline relationship than an offline affair. Drawing from Klein's work we have made the claim here that splitting is easier with an online affair compared to an offline affair, where the object of one's affections in face-to face encounters are more real than apparent.

REFERENCES

Atwood, J. D. (2002). Cyber-sex: The new affair treatment considerations. *Journal of Couple & Relationship Therapy, 3*(1), 37-56.

Betzig, L. (1989). Causes of conjugal dissolution: A cross cultural study. *Current Anthropology, 30,* 654-676.

Bollas, C. (1987) *The shadow of the object: Psychoanalysis of the unthought known.* London: Free Association Books.

Buss, D. M., & Shackelford, T. K. (1997). Susceptibility to infidelity in the first year of marriage. *Journal of Research in Personality, 31,* 193-221.

Carr, A. (1997). Terrorism of the couch–a psychoanalytic reading of the Oklahoma disaster and its aftermath. *Disaster Prevention and Management, 6*(1), 22-32.

Civin, M. A. (2000). *Male, female, e-mail: The struggle for relatedness in a paranoid society.* New York: Other Press.

Cooper, A. (1998). Sexuality and the Internet: Surfing its way into the new millennium. *CyberPsychology and Behavior, 1*(2), 24-28.

Fitness, J. (2001). Betrayal, rejection, revenge, and forgiveness: An interpersonal script approach. In M. Leary (Ed.), *Interpersonal rejection* (pp. 73-103). New York: Oxford University.

Kitzinger, C., & Powell, D. (1995). Engendering infidelity: Essentialist and social constructionist readings of a story completion task. *Feminism & Psychology, 5*(3), 345-372.

Klein, M. (1986). *The selected works of Melanie Klein* (J. Mitchell, Ed.). London, UK: Penguin Books.

Ogden, T. H. (1985). On Potential Space. *The International Journal of Psychoanalysis, 66,* 129-141.

Pittman, F. S., & Wagers, T. (1995). Crises of infidelity. In N. Jacobson & A. S. Gurman (Eds.), *Clinical handbook of couple therapy* (pp. 295-316). New York: Guilford.

Schwartz, H. (1990). *Narcissistic process and corporate decay: The theory of the organization ideal.* New York: New York University.

Whitty, M. T. (2003a). Pushing the wrong buttons: Men's and women's attitudes towards online and offline infidelity. *CyberPsychology & Behavior, 6*(6), 569-579.

Whitty, M. T. (2003b). Cyber-flirting: Playing at love on the Internet. *Theory and Psychology, 13*(3), 339-357.

Whitty, M. T. (2003c). The 'realness' of cyber-cheating: Men and women's representations of unfaithful Internet relationships. Manuscript submitted for publication.

Whitty, M. T., & Carr, A. N. (2003). Cyberspace as potential space: Considering the web as a playground to cyber-flirt. *Human Relations, 56*(7), 861-891.

Winnicott, D. W. (1997). *Playing and reality.* London: Tavistock. (Original work published 1971).

Yarab, P. E., Sensibaugh, C. C., & Allgeier, R. E. (1998). More than just sex: Gender differences in the incidence of self-defined unfaithful behavior in heterosexual dating relationships. *Journal of Psychology & Human Sexuality, 10*(2), 45-57.

Cyber-Affairs:
"What's the Big Deal?"
Therapeutic Considerations

Joan D. Atwood

SUMMARY. It can be estimated that 50-60% of married men and 45-55% of married women engage in extramarital sex at some time or another during their marriage and almost half come to therapy because of it. On-line infidelity accounts for a growing trend in reasons given for divorce according to the President of the American Academy of Matrimonial Lawyers and it is believed that it has been greatly underestimated. Because of the unfamiliarity and newness of this type of infidelity, mental health professionals are often unfamiliar with the dynamics associated with the concept of cyber-affairs and "virtual cheating." Many in fact do not consider the behavior as infidelity.

It is the purpose of this paper to explore this phenomenon, the cyber-affair, and examine the factors influencing it, the unique problems associated with this type of affair, along with a discussion of the therapeutic considerations. *[Article copies available for a fee from The Haworth Document Delivery Service: 1-800-HAWORTH. E-mail address: <docdelivery@ haworthpress.com> Website: <http://www.HaworthPress.com> ©2005 by The Haworth Press, Inc. All rights reserved.]*

Joan D. Atwood, PhD, is Director, Graduate Programs in Marriage and Family Therapy, Hofstra University, Hempstead, NY.

[Haworth co-indexing entry note]: "Cyber-Affairs: 'What's the Big Deal?' Therapeutic Considerations." Atwood, Joan D. Co-published simultaneously in *Journal of Couple & Relationship Therapy* (The Haworth Press) Vol. 4, No. 2/3, 2005, pp. 117-134; and: *Handbook of the Clinical Treatment of Infidelity* (ed: Fred P. Piercy, Katherine M. Hertlein, and Joseph L. Wetchler) The Haworth Press, Inc., 2005, pp. 117-134. Single or multiple copies of this article are available for a fee from The Haworth Document Delivery Service [1-800-HAWORTH, 9:00 a.m. - 5:00 p.m. (EST). E-mail address: docdelivery@haworthpress.com].

KEYWORDS. Infidelity, cyber-affairs, virtual cheating, cyber-flirting, cyber-sex

DEFINITION OF INTERNET INFIDELITY

In 2000, *The New York Times* reported that about one in four regular Internet users, or 21 million Americans, visited one of the more than 60,000 sex sites on the web at least once a month (Egan, 2000). It is not unreasonable to suspect that many of these individuals were in a couple relationship and that many of them engaged in chat-room activities (Schneider, 2001). It is difficult to define the cyber-affair just as it is difficult to define infidelity in the non-cyber world (Atwood & Seifer, 1997). Internet infidelity in this paper is described as an infidelity that consists of taking energy of any sort (thoughts, feelings, and behaviors) outside of the committed relationship in such a way that it damages interactions between the couple and negatively impacts the intimacy in the relationship. This is based on the assumption that anything that is deliberately hidden from a partner can create an emotional distance that could present a serious problem in the relationship (Shaw, 1997).

Lusterman (1998) defines infidelity as the breach of trust. He states that one significant element of the mutual trust in a marriage is the unspoken vow that the couple will remain sexually exclusive. Another is that there is a certain level of emotional intimacy that is reserved for the couple, not to be shared with others. Pittman and Pittman-Wagers (1995) agree and state that secrecy is a primary factor in the definition of infidelity. Infidelity then depends a great deal on the couple's understanding of the contract they have with one another and additionally when they define that contract as being threatened.

Internet infidelity is different from other traditional infidelities in that it appears to be anonymous and relatively safe, as it can be pursued in the privacy of one's own home or office. One's identity can be completely obscured or misrepresented. It can also be pursued any time, day or night with not much effort, seemingly not interfering with the individual's day to day living. Thus, some of the "signs" that a person is engaging in Internet infidelity would be: going to the computer in the middle of the night when everyone is sleeping, an escalation of time spent on the computer, demand for privacy, lying about computer activities, lack of interest in communicating with spouse, sexually or otherwise, unavailability to children because of computer activities, sudden additional time spent at work, etc.

When two people interact over the Internet, the conversation generally offers unconditional support and comfort. This electronic bond can offer the fantasy of the excitement, romance, and passion that may be missing in the current relationship. Instead of dealing with how to confront the issues of conflict in the marriage, the individuals use the cyber-relationship as an easy escape from the "real" issues. The Internet infidelity can become a means of coping with unresolved issues or unexpressed anger toward a partner as an outside person electronically offers understanding and comfort for hurt feelings (Young, O'Mara, & Buchanan, 1999).

TYPES OF INTERNET INFIDELITY

Like traditional infidelity, there are various types of cyber-relationships. Cooper, Putnam, Planchon and Bois (1999) divided cyber-sex users into three categories: recreational users, "at risk" users, and sexually compulsive users. Recreational users accessed on-line sexual connections out of curiosity; sexually compulsive users spent at least 11 hours per week online engaged in cyber-sex activities; at risk persons were persons who had no prior history of sexual on-line activity yet when afforded the opportunity and the time spend substantial time and energy on-line engaged in cyber-sex activities. Internet infidelity is based primarily on the extent of the interaction and the emotional commitment of the Surfer (the spouse committing the Internet infidelity) gives to the Internet and his or her cyber-friends. The continuum of involvement extends from simple curiosity, which is characteristic of most adults, to obsessive involvement, more characteristic of sex or relationship addicts.

When the subtle power, instant gratification and almost universal wish to be found interesting, attractive, and desirable come together, the unsuspecting user may find him or herself in a rapidly accelerating relationship with a momentum and life of its own.

The Cyber-Flirt (Chatting in Cyber-Space)

The Cyber-Flirt is a surfer who logs on to the Internet to chat with cyber-friends. The interactions can be on-line chats taking place in chat rooms, newsgroups, or IM's (instant messages). This type of interaction can become a problem for the couple when the Surfer goes on to the Internet to chat with the cyber-friends instead of spending time with his or her spouse or if the Cyber-Flirt begins telling marital problems to the cyber-friend.

The Cyber-Flirt is similar to Pittman and Pittman-Wagers' (1995) "Accidental Infidelity." These affairs are not expected, familiar, or predictable. Their participants did not seek each other out. They happened unexpectedly, by chance, even carelessly, with no real consideration of the consequence (Pittman & Pittman-Wagers, 1995, p. 301).

The danger is that the "harmless" on-line flirting interactions appear to become far more intense more quickly. Direct and explicit comments regarding sexual behavior can create a hyper stimulating effect and easily cross the line between innocent flirting and overt sexual interaction.

The progression between flirting and sexuality can become accelerated and the typical warning signals that alert one to infidelity can go unrecognized in cyber-space. Flirting suggests a limit or boundary embedded within. In cyber-space these usual markers are absent. The nonverbal signs of discomfort, smiles, and/or laughter are not available. Instead, an amorphous, uncharted, psychosocial vacuum exists which offers no resistance to the imaginative sexual impulses. In these cases, flirting can rapidly escalate to overt sexual interaction with little awareness on the parts of either member of the couple (Greenfield & Cooper, 1994, p. 1) and can thus threaten the couple's relationship.

Cyber-Sex

In this case, cyber-sex is defined when the surfer goes on the Internet to achieve sexual satisfaction, rather than gaining sexual satisfaction from his or her partner. The continuum of involvement extends from having casual cyber-sex with users in sex chat rooms and sexual websites to intimate sexual relations with one particular user. In addition, Schnarch (1997) believes that sex on the Internet is more like having an affair than having an ongoing relationship. "People often do things with less important partners, or when they are anonymous, that they cannot self-validate with a familiar significant spouse" (p. 18). Some seek outlets for their eroticism on-line in ways that they cannot validate and maintain in their primary relationship. They seek gratification thinking they are not jeopardizing their relationship.

The Cyber-Affair

The Cyber-Affair is defined as when one partner shares an emotional connection with one participating cyber-friend on the Internet. They use a great deal of their time thinking about each other and writing to each other. In this case, the cyber-couple is deeply involved. They may even take the relationship a step further and talk on the phone. This may or may not involve cyber-sex. Often it does. If the couple lives relatively close to each other, they may decide to meet. Even if they are geographically far apart, they may decide to meet. As Lusterman (1998) points out, an affair takes place over time. It may be very emotionally intense, and it may or may not involve sexual intercourse. "In a committed relationship if there is a secret sexual and/or romantic involvement outside of the relationship, it's experienced as an infidelity" (Lusterman, 1998, p. 18). Pittman and Pittman-Wagers (1995) state that romantic experience tends to occur at point of transition in people's lives, and it can serve the purpose of distracting them from having to change and adapt to new circumstances or a new stage of development. "Romance is an escape from too much reality; it is running away into fantasyland. It resembles a manic episode" (Pittman & Pittman-Wagers, 1995, p. 304).

FACTORS INFLUENCING INTERNET INFIDELITY

Listed below are six potential factors that are related or set the stage for Internet infidelity.

Cyber-Infidelity Is Anonymous

The anonymity associated with electronic communication allows the surfer to feel more open and free in talking with other users. The privacy of the cyber-space allows the surfer to share intimate feelings often reserved for a significant other. This may open the door to potential cyber-affair. Anonymity allows the surfer a greater sense of perceived control over the content, tone, and nature of the on-line experience. The person who is shy, obese, bald, etc., is transformed into Prince Charming in this electronic anonymous world. The surfer can create his or her own social conventions and define his or her own ground rules for social and sexual interaction. It allows the surfer to secretly engage in erotic chats with little or no fear of being caught by his or her spouse (Cooper, 2002).

The Cyber-Surfer Projects an Ideal Mate

When reading a typed message, there is a strong tendency to project–sometimes unconsciously–one's own expectations, wishes, anxieties and/or fears into what the person wrote. There is a high possibility of the surfer distorting the person's intended meaning. It is possible that perhaps all computer transference involves a blending of the user's mind with the "cyber-space" created by the machine. Cyber-space is indeed a psychological space, an extension of the user's intrapsychic world. Computers create a transitional space–an intermediate zone between self and other–where identifications, partial identifications, internalization and introjects interact with each other. This can explain how users react to other people they encounter in cyber-space. Communicating only by typed text in e-mail, chat rooms and newsgroups results in a highly ambiguous environment. The other person is not seen or heard–they are a shadowy figure, a screen or backdrop onto which any variety of transference reactions can be launched (Suler, 1998).

Cyber-Infidelity Often Attracts Those with Intimacy Issues

There are situations whereby persons may seek out romantic partners but be emotionally unable to handle the pressures of relationships once formed. These types of individuals may have problems with intimacy and/or fear vulnerability. Internet infidelity indicates that a surfer might be developed enough emotionally to find a partner but perhaps not developed enough to be intimate and open in the relationship with that partner.

> He or she might be partially separated, incompletely individuated or mostly undifferentiated. Separation begins with the realization that one is a separate person from mother and eventually from all others. Individuation develops as a child or adult finally assumes and places value on their own individual characteristics. (Shaw, 1997, p. 31)

Schnarch (1991) states in *The Sexual Crucible* that motivation without differentiation leads to more affairs than "marital reconstruction" (p. 371). Basically, it is difficult for marriage to compete with the Internet. He states that the level of differentiation is an important determinant of the likelihood of it emerging in Internet infidelity. The impact of the infidelity is usually multisystemic, offering the surfer:

> (1) defiance of feeling controlled and dominated by the spouse; (2) gratification of the desire to punish, deprive, hurt or get one up on the spouse; (3) avoidance of intimacy in the marriage while

appearing to seek (or find) it on the Internet, and (4) use of the affair as a strategic buffer in the marriage and vice versa. (Schnarch, 1991, p. 367)

He believes that at low levels of differentiation, monogamy results from "reciprocal extortion of sexual exclusivity" (p. 372). This lose-lose contact fertilizes common unresolved autonomy issues that bloom into control fights and rebellious affairs. In highly differentiated couples, "the monogamy is based on two unilateral commitments for which partners owe each other nothing (except perhaps respect). The covenant is not made to the partner but rather to oneself, with the partner as witness and secondary beneficiary" (Schnarch, 1991, p. 372).

Cyber-Infidelity Regulates Anxiety

In any relationship, anxiety may arise as the individuals attempt to balance their need for closeness with their need for autonomy (Bowen, 1978). The greater the fusion of the couple, the more difficult the task of finding a stable balance satisfying to both. The resulting anxiety over regulating closeness and distance can result in triangulation. Triangulation involves a situation where emotional energy is invested in a third person, place, or thing. This investment of energy could involve work, golf, a child, an affair, or the Internet. The Internet may provide companionship, sexual fulfillment, tenderness and/or adventure. In this sort of triangulation, there is a tacit or covert agreement (sometimes even overt) by the couple to manage their anxiety by means of the Internet (Bowen, 1978).

The main attraction of the Internet is the whole notion of emotional contact without risk, exposure, or being known. This is accomplished because the cyber-affair offers romantic contact while keeping "the partner from becoming a pivotal figure in one's life" (Schnarch, 1997, p. 17). Shaw (1997) believes that it is possible that the cyber-affair is resultant from the couple's underdeveloped relational skills. Their poor survival patterns help them avoid confronting their loneliness and other issues in the relationship because they can consciously withdraw from each other at any time. The call of the Internet so as to avoid confronting disappointment and conflict can be irresistible.

Cyber-Infidelity Becomes a Source of Communication

The Internet can decrease the chance of the surfer to share meaning with his or her spouse. It can prevent clear, direct, person-centered communication. Instead of communicating feelings to one's spouse, the surfer tends to transfer his or her emotions on to the user(s) in cyberspace. Internet infidelity can be a result of the couple's inability to communicate feelings or needs to one another. It also can indicate that the couple does not have the verbal skills to solve problems together, or be able to accommodate to one another's needs or interests.

Cyber-Infidelity Addiction

Young (1999) defines Internet addiction as an impulse-control disorder, which does not involve an intoxicant. She found that serious relationship problems were reported by fifty-three percent of the cyberaddicts surveyed. Addicts gradually spend less time with the people in their lives in exchange for solitary time in front of the computer. Marriages appear to be the most affected as Internet use interferes with the marital and family responsibilities and obligations. In these cases, individuals may form online relationships, which over time can replace time spent with the spouse and/or children. The addicted spouse tends to socially isolate him or herself and may refuse to engage in typical events once enjoyed by the couple such as going out to dinner, traveling, or seeing a movie. Instead, they prefer on-line companions (Young, 1999). The ability to carry out romantic and sexual relationships on-line further then deteriorates the stability of the real life couple. As the spouse exerts more pressure on the surfer to interact, the surfer may continue to emotionally and socially withdraw from the marriage, exerting more effort to maintain the recently discovered on-line "lovers."

THERAPEUTIC CONSIDERATIONS

Couples who come for therapy with the issue of Internet infidelity are experiencing problems in their relationship. They have attempted many solutions, which have been unsuccessful. Once the infidelity is out in the open, couples tend to feel ambivalent, harboring both negative and positive feelings toward the person, thing, or situation. They also tend to experience combinations of devastation, hurt, betrayal, loss of self-esteem, mistrust, suspicion, fear, anger, distrust, and blame. At times extreme responses may occur such as physical abuse or suicide attempts. In some cases, the spouse begins to doubt his or her judgement and even sanity, as a strange form of "gaslighting" occurs where the non-surfer spouse may question the validity of his or her complaints, feeling that, "after all the cyber-relationship is not really real." The term "Gaslighting" has been coined as a metaphor for the "head games" which occurred in the classic movie *Gaslight,* starring Charles Boyer and Ingrid Bergman. In the film, the husband systematically attempts to drive his wife mad by having the gaslights flicker and convincing his wife that she is imagining these events. It is only after the intervention of a Scotland Yard detective that her perceptions are validated and she realizes the full implications of her husband's plot to deceive her. What sometimes occurs when an affair is uncovered is that the accused attempts to convince his or her spouse that s/he has imagined many of the incidents and/or misinterpreted the evidence. There is not only an attempt to conceal with regard to gaslighting but an attempt to falsify information as well (Maheu & Subotnik, 2001).

It is at this point that the gaslighting begins to become destructive, as more and more evidence of the affair is met with more assertions of the spouse's "wild imagination." One might recall that Sullivan and Swick (1968) defined reality as that which can be consensually validated. In the case of a denied affair, the only person who could possibly validate one's perceptions will not confirm what the individual "knows" s/he heard or saw. As a matter of fact, s/he is, at times, told that s/he is "hearing things" or imagining them, reinforcing the notion s/he might actually be "losing his or her mind." Often in the initial stages of the Internet infidelity, the non-surfer spouse may become suspicious of the surfer's time spent on the Internet and the resulting dismissal of other areas of his or her life. Frequently the surfer becomes edgy, short with the children, and generally seems preoccupied. This may cause the non-surfer spouse to become suspicious of his or her suspicions and discount them, only to experience them again when the surfer spouse withdraws or spends time on the computer. The non-surfer spouse often feels like s/he is on an emotional rollercoaster.

Evaluation

According to Cooper et al. (1999), the therapist needs to first determine to what extent is the surfer's interaction on the Internet. Access, affordability and anonymity provided by the Internet could transform simpler, more common relational difficulties into more complex and serious troubles (Cooper et al., 1999). Once the assessment of the individual's or couple's on-line activities is accomplished, detailed information about the meanings and effects of the activities could be explored. The therapist could examine how many hours are spent on-line, what the level of direct activity is on the Internet, what type of infidelity, and how severe it is. It is also helpful to examine the intrapsychic roots of their behavior as well as current life circumstances that maintain it. Cooper, Putnam, Planchon, and Boies (1999) found that the amount of time spent on-line in sexual activities was highly correlated with the degree to which life problems were reported (see also Maheu & Subotnik, 2001b).

In addition, it would be helpful if the therapist explored also the intimate and sexual part of the couple's relationship (Schneider, 2002, as cited in Cooper, 2002). In many cases, the surfer spouse has substituted cyber-sex for sex with his or her partner. Many spouses report that the surfer spouse had withdrawn his sexuality, intimacy and attention from the family. It is important to also explore gender differences in terms of the meanings and reasons given by the couple for Cyber-Infidelity. It is probably true that more men visit pornography sites; whereas more women visit chat rooms. Women tend to be more relational in their interactions and thus would pursue Cyber-Relationships more so than Cyber-Sex, although one may easily lead to the other (Maheu & Subotnik, 2001; Young, 2001).

Crisis Intervention

Infidelity often presents itself in the midst of crisis, with the participants experiencing emotions that seem overwhelming and out of control. The first step then is providing an emergency response. "Until the infidelity is revealed, the marriage and the therapy are merely subterfuge" (Pittman & Pittman-Wagers, 1995, p. 308). It is helpful if the therapist can provide a calm, safe setting in which the surfer and the spouse can sit down facing each other and examine what has occurred. The therapist conveys confidence that the couple will be able to accomplish this. The therapist also communicates to the couple that people can and do work through infidelity and that it does not necessarily signal the end of the relationship. In so doing, the couple can see that there are options and that drastic measures may not be necessary. "Optimism about infidelity requires the therapist to get everyone to focus on the behavior, which is controllable, rather than the emotions, which seem overwhelming and out of control" (Pittman & Pittman-Wagers, 1995, p. 311).

Loss of Self-Esteem

Cyber-infidelity chips away at the partner's self-esteem (Spring, 1996). S/he simply cannot compete with the "perfect" fantasy person. In therapy one wife wondered, "When he closes his eyes when we make love, what is he thinking or visualizing? Is he picturing his cyber-sex goddess or is he thinking about me in my chubby body?" She reported that these thoughts limited her abilities to respond sexually to him.

Facing the Trauma of the Act: It IS a "Big Deal!"

Many surfer spouses do not feel that cyber-infidelity is a "big deal." In fact, the surfer spouse may deny that cyber-infidelity is an affair. S/he may feel that there was no "real" body contact that took place and that they did not actually engage in sex with the person. The spouses, on the other hand, often feel traumatized and along with feeling hurt and angry often worry about escalation of the cyber-sex into "real" contact and do consider the act as adultery and "cheating." There is some basis to their fears as Cooper et al. (1999) and Cooper et al. (2000) point out, accessing sex on the Internet has the potential to escalate preexisting sex addiction as well as to create new disorders.

It is crucially important for therapists not to underestimate the adverse consequences of the cyber-sex behavior. Some common mistakes made by therapists in these situations are to (1) encourage the partner to be more accepting of the surfer spouses' activities, (2) to label the surfer spouse as having sexual disinterest, (3) to believe that the behavior is not "really" sex, and/or (4) not to assess the meaning of the behavior for both spouses.

Loss of the Cyber-Lover

Loss of the cyber-lover is another issue at this time. Over the numerous e-mails, the cyber-person has become an important confidante in the surfer's life and the abrupt cessation of this relationship (which must happen if the marriage is to go forward) can cause much pain and sorrow. It is imperative that the surfer stops the behavior, both the infidelity and the lying. Anything that is deliberately hidden from a partner (whether it is the fact of being involved in an on-line affair or the specifics of the on-line interactions) creates an emotional distance that can present a serious problem that is difficult to overcome. This decision to stop the Internet infidelity is best if it arises from the couple and not be a dictum of the therapist. It is also important that before continuing in the therapy that the surfer and the spouse affirm their commitment to the marriage.

Dealing with Underlying Issues

Engaging both spouses in an examination process is an important step toward dealing with Internet infidelity. To make sense of the infidelity, it is helpful if the partners explore the secrets in their relationship, what they mean and why they feel that hiding a portion of the self is necessary. The partners need to explore unresolved issues (if any) that fuel intellectual power struggles and relentless transference behaviors–both current and historical. In this way they can reclaim their projections. "The ultimate challenge of integrity is to be fully and uninhibitedly one self with one's partner rather than on-line with a stranger" (Shaw, 1997, p. 33).

It is important for the surfer spouse to examine issues of self-presentation (i.e., presenting yourself the way you want to be seen rather than how you actually are) when considering the merits of Internet infidelity (Schnarch, 1997). Does the surfer present him/her self differently on the Internet from his/ her "real" relationship? Why does the surfer have difficulty showing that side of his/her self in the relationship? What are the surfer's needs that are met in the cyber-relationship that are not met in the marital relationship? How can the non-surfer spouse help to create an atmosphere of teamwork and safety so that honesty can prevail?

Build Communication

Cyber-sex takes the surfer partner away from his or her partner in terms of sexuality, attention, emotion, and communication. It is also important to consider these effects on the children. For example, it is probably true that the surfer spouse is less available to spend time with his or her children, and in extreme cases, there might be a failure to fulfill family responsibilities (see Schneider, 2000b). One fifteen year client came into therapy very distraught reporting that she had just learned her father was visiting porn sites. She had gone on the computer after he had used it and went into the history menu.

The focus of the therapy should be on empowerment and team building. This occurs through communication. There is a focus on the behaviors and communications that permit each member of the marital unit to earn each other's trust and respect. Anger must be diffused through healthy ventilation within the sessions and in the couple's home life. Guilt must be addressed, both the guilt of the surfer about what s/he has done and that of the nonparticipating spouse about what s/he may have contributed to the breakdown of the couple's system. At this point, the therapist could help the couple resolve their intensely ambivalent feelings about each other so that the marriage can go forward (Nichols, 1988).

Restoration of open communication and deepening of understanding of the current meaning or meanings of the cyber-affair are crucial. This may include determining what the partners know and what they wish to know about the affair, as well as the meaning it holds for each (Nichols, 1988, p. 193). Restoration of communication also includes dealing with what is known and acknowledged by both spouses, what is (was) the meaning of the interaction on the Internet to each of the marital partners and their marriage, and a damage control assessment.

In this phase, the therapist could emphasize changing the rules of communication, taking great care to ensure that both partners feel heard and validated. A way to do so is by filtering out several troublesome kinds of communications, such as blame (attributing bad intentions or bad traits to another or oneself), invalidation (undercutting the other person's confidence in his or her own feelings and perceptions), stalemating (closing down the possibilities for the relationship or either partner to change, and vagueness (general words or phrases that lend themselves to misinterpretations or misunderstandings) (O'Hanlon & Hudson, 1994, p. 161).

Once the couple's communication improves, it is important for them to recognize that trust may remain as an issue, regardless of the understanding of the meaning of the infidelity involvement. At some point in the therapy, it is important and helpful if the couple can create a ritual to put the past Internet infidelity in perspective. They could write out their feelings in a notebook and then perhaps include some of the e-mail symbolic of the affair. They can place the materials in shoebox and then bury the shoebox in their backyard–a symbolic burying of the past if you will. Couples should design the ritual themselves and they should decide when it should occur. The only rule is that once they have buried the past, they cannot dig it up again symbolically meaning that they may no longer discuss the Internet infidelity.

Rebuilding Marital Trust

In the initial stages of therapy, it is suggested that simple solutions be considered. Love Addicts Anonymous suggest moving the computer to an open area, not using the Internet, using the computer only for planned, specified tasks, being on-line when family members are around, adding Internet control tools, and arranging for some sort of accountability if there is Internet access at work (Delmonico, Griffin, & Berg, 2002, in Cooper, 2002).

Lusterman (1998) believes that honesty is the necessary prelude to trust and that trust is the prelude to intimacy. Internet infidelity often happens inside the couple's home and the surfer's behavior is centralized around the computer, a tool that may also be used for non-romantic purposes such as business or home finances. In this sense the betrayal of the marriage may seem more intense as the non-surfer may feel that s/he is sleeping with the cyber-partner in their marital home so to speak. However, each time the surfer approaches the computer for a legitimate reason. It may trigger feelings of suspicion and jealousy for the spouse. The therapist can help the couple to evaluate how the computer will be used at home so that they can establish reasonable ground rules such as supervised computer use or moving the computer into a public area of the family home until a stronger trust base is built (Young, 1999). The surfer spouse must facilitate trust in the partner and the partner has to work on believing that there is a commitment to the marriage.

It is important to help the spouses understand the motives leading up to the Internet infidelity. The surfer may rationalize the behavior as just fantasy, typed words on a screen, or say that cyber-sex is not cheating because of the lack of physical contact. This is a form of "gaslighting" and can serve to "crazy-make" the non-surfer spouse because his or her reality is being invalidated. It is important for the therapist to focus on ways for the surfer to take responsibility for his/her actions (Young, 1999). In so doing, the therapist should take a benevolent stance rather than a judgmental one.

Here the therapist could help the couple evaluate how the Internet infidelity has hurt the relationship and help formulate relationship enhancing goals that can assist them in renewing their commitment so that intimacy can grow once again. The therapist can ask about the couple's activity pre-Internet cyber-relationship. How did they have fun then? What were the types of activities the couple did before the Internet came into their lives? The couple could develop a couple contract where they spend time together as a couple where they are free of distraction and where they can be honest, loving, and caring toward each other.

Constructing New Stories

The stories we create about our lives and relationships both arise from and shape our experiences. Our many life stories are both our creations and our creators. They are the principal way that each of us participates with others in the making and remaking of ourselves as social beings. When partners are at an impasse in their relationship, their individual and couple stories have become predominantly narratives of limitation. The past is experienced as fixed and foreclosed rather than in flux and open (Atwood, 1997; Roth & Chasin, 1994).

During this phase the therapist can help the couple become more aware that they have a choice in change. They can see that that there are numerous scripts to choose from. Change requires at least a two-sided perspective, and a therapist may seek to construct a relational definition by assisting the couple in uncovering two or more complementary definitions of the problem. Here, complementary questions can be introduced to help deconstruct the dominant explanation and to assist couples in achieving a relational or double description of the problem. This double description then provides the source of new responses (Atwood & Seifer, 1997).

Future focus enables the couple to visualize their relationship in which the Internet infidelity is no longer an issue and the couple feels empowered and confident that they possess skills necessary to solve other problems. By asking questions about future trends and choices, the therapist is making that future more real and more stable.

Ritual for a Fresh Start

At the end of the therapy, a ritual for a fresh start may be helpful. At this time, couples can choose a new anniversary date when they recommit to each other. They can rewrite their marital vows and hold a ceremony where they "remarry" each other. They can purchase new wedding rings. "Along with restating their commitment to each other and to the relationship, they can write down their future relationship vision. This becomes their future image, the template for their relationship" (Atwood & Seifer, 1997, p. 71).

CONCLUSIONS

Internet infidelity is a new and increasing problem couples are bringing into therapy. In these cases, the therapist's role in helping the couple is first to explore the therapist's own feelings about Internet infidelity–does the therapist consider it a breach of the couple contract? Does the therapist consider it infidelity? Next it is helpful to evaluate the extent of the infidelity, and to provide a crisis intervention for the couple. Here the couple can explore their feelings about the Internet infidelity, ultimately putting it in perspective. Once there is a calm and safe setting, the therapist could examine how the Internet provided the couple with an excuse not to relate to one another. Feelings of mistrust, loss of self-esteem, and the hurt and anger could be explored and validated. For the spouse, Internet infidelity is a big deal. Once the couple is able to move beyond the infidelity, the therapist could work on building the couple's communication and trust with each other, assisting them to construct new stories about their future. At the end of therapy the couple should feel empowered in their skills and enhanced as a team–stronger for having conquered the affair.

Internet infidelity has become a growing trend faced by many couples therapists. Unlike traditional infidelity, Internet infidelity often occurs in one's home or office, sometimes with no real thought of looking for an affair. Like traditional infidelity, Internet infidelity could be an indicator that there are issues in the relationship that need to be addressed. This paper focused on this new phenomenon, examined some of the factors often associated with this type of infidelity and explored some therapeutic considerations.

REFERENCES

Atwood, J. D. (Ed.) (1997). *Challenging family therapy situations: Perspectives in social construction*. New York: Springer.

Atwood, J. D., & Seifer, M. (1997). Extramarital affairs and constructed meaning: A social constructionist therapeutic approach. *American Journal of Family Therapy*, *25*(1), 55-75.

Cooper, A., Putnam, D., Planchon, L., & Boies, S. (1999). On-line sexual compulsivity: Getting tangled in the net. *Sexual Addiction and Compulsivity*, *6*(2), 79-201.

Cooper, A., Delmonico, D., & Burg, R. (2000). Cybersex users, abusers, and compulsives. New findings and implications. *Sexual Addiction & Compulsivity*, *7*(1), 5-30.

Cooper, A. (2002). *Sex and the internet: A guidebook for clinicians*. New York: Brunner-Routledge.

Egan, T. (2000). Wall Street meets pornography. *New York Times*. [On-line]. Available: http://www.nytimes.com/2000/10/23/technology/23PORN.html

Glover, C., & Redshaw, I. B. (1996). *Locus of control among internet users: A preliminary investigation of the internet* [On-line]. Available: http://pegasus.cc.ucf.edu/~cwg65985/results.html

Greenfield, D. N., & Cooper, A. (1994). *Crossing the line–On line*. [On-line]. Available: http://www.shpm.com/articles/cyber_romance/sexcross.html

Hamman, R. B. (1996). The role of fantasy in the construction of the online other: A selection of interviews and participant observations from cyber-space. [On-line]. Available: http://www.socio.demon.co.uk/fantasy.html

Hudson-O'Hanlon, W., & O'Hanlon-Hudson, P. (1994). Co-authoring a love story: Solution-oriented marital therapy. In M. F. Hoyt (Ed.), *Constructive therapies*. New York: Guilford Press.

Humphrey, F. G. (1987). Treating extramarital sexual relationships in sex and couples therapy. In G. R. Weeks & L. Hof (Eds.), *Integrating sex and marital therapy: A clinical guide*. New York: Brunner/Mazel.

Katz, J. E., & Aspden, P. (1998). Friendship formation in cyber-space: Analysis of a national survey of users. [On-line]. Available: http:// http://www.nicoladoering.net/Hogrefe/katz.htm

Leiblum, S. R. (1997). Sex and the net: Clinical implications. *Journal of Sex Education & Therapy, 22*(1), 15-20.

Lusterman, D. (1998). *Infidelity: A survival guide*. New York: MJF Books.

Maheu, M., & Subotnik, R. (2001). *Infidelity on the internet*. CA: Sourcebook Trade.

Mahler, M. S., Pine, F., & Bergman, A. (1975). *The psychological birth of the human infant: Symbiosis and individuation*. New York: Basic Books.

Nichols, W. C. (1988). *Marital therapy: An integrative approach*. New York: Guilford Press.

Parks, M. R., & Floyd, K. (1996). Making friends in cyber-space. *Journal of Communication, 46*(1), 80-97.

Pittman, F. S., & Pittman Wagers, T. (1995). Crises of infidelity. In N. Jacobson & A. Gurman (Eds.), *Clinical handbook of couple therapy*. New York: Guilford Press.

Quittner, J. (1997). Divorce Internet style. *Time,* April 14, p. 72.

Roth, S., & Chasin, R. (1994). Entering one another's worlds of meaning and imagination: Dramatic enactment and narrative couple therapy. In M. F. Hoyt (Ed.), *Constructive therapies*. New York: Guilford Press.

Schnarch, D. (1991). *Constructing the sexual crucible: An integration of sexual and marital therapy*. New York: W. W. Norton & Co.

Schnarch, D. (1997). Sex, intimacy, and the internet. *Journal of Sex Education & Therapy, 22*(1), 15-20.

Schneider, J. (2000a). A qualitative study of cyber-sex participants: Gender differences, recovery issues, and implications for therapists. *Sexual Addiction and Compulsivity, 7*, 249-278.

Schneider, J. (2000b). Effects of cyber-sex, addiction on the family: Results of a survey. *Sexual Addiction and Compulsivity, 7*(1), 31-58.

Sempsey, J. (1997). *Psyber Psychology: A Literature review Pertaining to the Psycho/Social Aspects of Multi-User Dimensions in Cyber-Space.* [On-line]. Available: http://journal.tinymush.org/v2n1/sempsey.html

Shaw, J. (1997) Treatment rationale for Internet infidelity. *Journal of Sex Education and Therapy, 22*(1), 29-34.

Suler, J. (1997). *The final showdown between in-person and cyber-space relationships.* [On-line]. Available: http://www.rider.edu/users/suler/psycyber/showdown.html.

Suler, J. (1998). *Mom, Dad, Computer (Transference Reactions to Computers).* [On-line]. Available: http://www.rider.edu/users/suler/psycyber/comptransf.html

Sullivan, H., & Swick, H. (1968). *The interpersonal theory of psychiatry.* New York: W. W. Norton & Co.

Thompson, A. T. (1983). Extramarital sex: A review of research literature. *Journal of Sex Research, 19*(1), 1-22.

Turkle, S. (1995). *Life on the screen: Identity in the age of the Internet.* New York: Simon and Schuster.

Vaughan, P. (1998). *On-line Affairs.* [On-line]. Available: http:// www.vaughan-vaughan.com/com010.html

Young, K. (1996). *Internet addiction: The emergence of a new clinical disorder.* Paper presented at the 104th annual meeting of the American Psychological Association, August 11, 1996. Toronto, Canada.

Young, K. (1999). Internet addiction: Symptoms, evaluation and treatment. In L. VandeCreek & T. Jackson (Eds.), *Innovations in clinical practice: A source book.* Sarasota, FL: Professional Resource Press.

Young, K., O'Mara, J., & Buchanan, J. (1999). *Cybersex and infidelity On-line: Implications for evaluation and treatment.* Poster presented at the 107th annual meeting of the American Psychological Association. August 21, 1999. Hynes Convention Center.

Young, K. (2001). *Tangled in a web: Understanding cybersex from fantasy to addiction.* Bloomington, IN: First Books Library.

The Relationship, If Any, Between Marriage and Infidelity

Frank S. Pittman III
Tina Pittman Wagers

SUMMARY. Infidelity has been hypothesized to be caused by any number of factors, including unhappy marriages. The current article explores the myths about infidelity and its treatment. Advice is offered to those treating affairs, and to those interested in successful marriages. *[Article copies available for a fee from The Haworth Document Delivery Service: 1-800-HAWORTH. E-mail address: <docdelivery@haworthpress.com> Website: <http://www.HaworthPress.com> © 2005 by The Haworth Press, Inc. All rights reserved.]*

Frank S. Pittman III, MD, is affiliated with Northside Hospital Doctors Centre, 960 Johnson Ferry Road, Northeast, Suite 543, Atlanta, GA 30342 (E-mail: FSP3MD@aol.com).

Tina Pittman Wagers, MSW, PsyD, is affiliated with the Department of Psychology, University of Colorado at Boulder, 345 UCB, Boulder, CO 80309-0345 (E-mail: Tina@Wagers.net).

[Haworth co-indexing entry note]: "The Relationship, If Any, Between Marriage and Infidelity." Pittman III, Frank S, and Tina Pittman Wagers. Co-published simultaneously in *Journal of Couple & Relationship Therapy* (The Haworth Press) Vol. 4, No. 2/3, 2005, pp. 135-148; and: *Handbook of the Clinical Treatment of Infidelity* (ed: Fred P. Piercy, Katherine M. Hertlein, and Joseph L. Wetchler) The Haworth Press, Inc., 2005, pp. 135-148. Single or multiple copies of this article are available for a fee from The Haworth Document Delivery Service [1-800-HAWORTH, 9:00 a.m. - 5:00 p.m. (EST). E-mail address: docdelivery@haworthpress.com].

Available online at http://www.haworthpress.com/web/JCRT
© 2005 by The Haworth Press, Inc. All rights reserved.
doi:10.1300/J398v04n02_12

KEYWORDS. Infidelity, marriage, monogamy, myths, treatment

Affairs drive people crazy. Infidelity and the fear of its revelation confuse, disorient, and emotionally overload participants, bystanders, and observers, even therapists. The cultural and therapeutic myths about infidelity, its causes, and its treatment further confound the situation. It seems absurd that something so common is so badly misunderstood.

Affairs are prevalent, in good marriages and in bad, but are not the norm for either men or women. Glass and Wright (1992) reported that 44% of married men and 25% of married women had at least one extramarital involvement. Their figures seem high because they include emotional affairs which were never actually consummated. Some estimates are even higher. One Chicago study (Michael, Gagnon, Laumann, & Kolata, 1994) found that 25% of men and 15% of women admitted having had extramarital sexual involvements. They projected that, if affairs are distributed randomly over the course of marriages, then half of husbands and a third of wives would eventually stray. (Of course, affairs are not distributed randomly over the course of a lifetime.) Still, infidelity is not the norm: most wives are faithful for a lifetime and most husbands are faithful most of the time.

Affairs create painful and unexpected consequences. Amato and Roberts (1997) report that infidelity is the most singularly identified problem that is correlated with divorce. Out of twelve thousand or so couples over a 40-year marriage therapy practice, I (FP) have seen less than a dozen established first marriages end in divorce without someone being unfaithful–and it is not the knowledge of an affair that blows the marriage apart. The ones most likely to end in post-affair divorce are those in which the infidel tried to keep it secret through the whole domestic disaster. *Affairs are the sine qua non of divorce.*

The hallmark of infidelity is not necessarily sex, but secrecy. Infidelity seems best defined as a betrayal of the couple's agreement about sexual involvement and romantic entanglement outside the marriage. Infidelity may involve activity, connections, attractions or even looking at pictures or typing messages to people on the internet. A couple's idiosyncratic boundaries may be influenced by families of origin, peers, culture, and gender expectations. The boundaries are not always clear. *"If you don't know whether what you are doing constitutes an affair or not, ask your spouse"* (Pittman, 1989).

A FEW CULTURAL MYTHS

How couples deal with boundary violations is influenced by cultural myths, forwarded by friends, family members, Dear Abby, and sometimes, therapists. Below are a few of these myths.

What They Don't Know Won't Hurt Them

In some circles, the conventional wisdom about infidelity is "Deny! Deny! Deny!" This is disastrous. The betrayal of infidelity is not as much in the illicit, furtive sex, or even the obsession with it, as in the lie and the inevitable distance that it creates. Intimacy is "knowing" and not knowing what your partner is doing destroys the intimacy of the marriage. The conventional wisdom has held that "what people don't know won't hurt them," that ignorance and disorientation of the betrayed spouse during an affair will offer safety, even if it destroys the intimacy of the marriage and keeps it from offering sanctuary, reality testing, or sanity. Stephen Sondheim, in his musical FOLLIES, has the wife of a philanderer sing "You said you loved me, but were you just being kind, or am I losing my mind?"

While secrecy may be comfortable in the short run, it is this same secrecy that eventually erodes intimacy and trust and provides a real hazard to rebuilding a marriage.

"My Marriage Wasn't Making Me Happy"

Infidelity occurs in happy and unhappy marriages alike, though infidelity has the potential to make a happy marriage unhappy pretty quickly. The notion that infidelity is caused by marital distress alone is so far unsupported by the data (Treas & Giesen, 2000) although marital distress may be part of the context of infidelity, especially for women. Glass and Wright (1992) report that only 30% of men who had been involved in infidelity reported marital distress before their affair, while 60% of women were unhappy before their affair. Similar findings are reported by Hunt (1969). However, these results are retrospective, and it may be that individuals who rate marital satisfaction after they have had an affair may have developed a post-hoc rationalization of why the affair occurred. Making external vs. internal attributions of problems has also been noted in people's post-hoc explanations of divorce (Amato & Rogers, 1997; Rasmussen & Ferraro, 1979). In cases of infidelity, betrayed spouses tend to blame marital problems on the infidelity, and infidels blame the infidelity on marital distress (Spanier & Margolis, 1983).

We know that women pay more attention to interpersonal relationships than men (Gilligan,1982). In their efforts to improve their relationships, they are more likely to find things that displease them. They are more likely to experience their unhappiness as caused by flawed relationships and more likely to seek couples' therapy than their husbands (Jacobson, Dobson, Fruzzetti, Schmaling, & Salusky, 1991). Women are also more likely to see their blissful affair as a way out of their "unhappy" marriage. In contrast, while men are at increased risk for depression when a marriage is disrupted, they may not attend to their relationship closely enough to notice or respond to interpersonal difficulties in the same way women do. Men may be less likely to blame their affairs on their marriage, but they are also less likely to see the impact of the affair on the marriage. They are certainly more likely to compartmentalize affairs and dismiss them as insignificant.

Whether marital distress was identified before the affair began or after it had been going for a while, some men and more women may retrospectively fault some relational flaw as they try to explain how they got into the affair. Even given the presence of distress in the relationship that precedes infidelity, *it would be absurd to view the affair as having been _caused_ by the distress, just as it would be outrageous to view abusive behavior or alcoholism as _caused_ by relationship distress.* Whatever the stresses of marriage, other individuals at the same decision point might have chosen to enter therapy, call a friend, communicate differently with their spouse, or start an exercise program. When someone has made the decision to have an affair, the decision making needs to be a focus of the treatment. The question is not "How did your husband or wife make you have the affair?" but "How did infidelity (or violence or getting drunk or suicide bombing) get into your repertoire of responses to stressful situations?"

Likewise, those who expect marriage to make them happy are missing the point. *Marriage is not supposed to make people happy; it is supposed to make people married,* so they don't have to date, and are thus free to lead productive, useful, gratifying lives.

But I'm in Love

If affair participants are inclined to view their marriages as dissatisfying, then the contrast to being "in love" with a new affair partner can prove a clear and present danger to the marriage.

Falling in love is a measurable biological state, akin to a manic episode or a bout of temporary insanity. It is overwhelming, like a neurochemical tidal wave, disorienting lives in ways that were not anticipated and can not be understood. Whether people enter affairs blindly or calculatedly, the neurochemistry of "being in love" is extraordinarily difficult to escape and produces an experience akin to withdrawal from an addictive drug.

Helen Fisher (1992), in *Anatomy of Love*, has explained the neurochemistry when human beings and other beasts fall in and out of love. Simply, the lust and attachment of pair bonding may start with the anticipation of sex, may trigger hefty squirts of amphetamines and testosterone, making the sufferer oversexed, intensely excited, and obsessed with the love object. At the same time, there is a drop in levels of oxytocin and vasopressin, the nurturing domestic hormones, so people who are going through the temporary insanity of falling in love may have little love to give outside that obsessive relationship, and may abandon or disregard children, mates, friends and family, and all the other loved ones of a lifetime. Interestingly, during these states of obsessive lust or in-loveness, serotonin levels drop and there is insecurity and panic at the thought of losing this new fantasy object. If the obsessive new relationship is socially sanctioned and makes the life of the lover more comfortable, the vasopressin and oxytocin will rise, the amphetamine and testosterone will settle down and the burgeoning serotonin will produce a state of mellow, blissful joy. If the new relationship costs too much and isolates the couple from other sources of support, it will gradually turn into an irritant and bother. As Cole Porter pointed out: "We should have been aware that our love affair was too hot not to cool down."

Unfortunately, falling in love with dangerous strangers, with its manic side effects, may be more thrilling than pre- or post-affair domesticity. Life in the real world may feel like a letdown after a flight to la-la-land. The contrast may leave the affair participant convinced that he or she is not "in-love" when the affair ends. Therapists and level headed bystanders have to understand and convey the reality that the neurochemistry of falling in love is not a predictor of the realities of long-term relationships. Being in-love is easy, for a while, and at its peak takes less work than marriage. But it is a helluva lot harder to clean up after.

TREATMENT MYTHS

Crises of infidelity, however stormy and messy and treacherous, are quite treatable and betrayed marriages quite salvageable. Glass (2003) agrees. The outcome depends, among other things, on the attitude, level of optimism and level of squeamishness of the therapist.

"This Marriage Was a Mistake"

Yet *the highly destructive conventional wisdom on the matter among marriage therapists and even in the marriage literature holds that infidelity is evidence that the marriage should never have happened,* that the couple married the wrong people and, presumably, rather than ending the affair the couple should end the marriage. Some marital therapists have posited that infidelity is nearly universal in marriage, and that it need not be mentioned in the therapeutic process of dismantling marriages eroded by complaints, criticism, contempt, or stonewalling.

There are immature people who can't tell the difference between mates and parents and expect their husband or wife to keep them faithful. They may even blame their partner if they themselves don't behave and screw up. "If this were the right marriage, and he or she were my real soulmate, I wouldn't be doing what I'm doing with this stranger, so it's not my fault. I just wasn't *really* in love." *It is strange how many people fail to know that if they want to feel more in love they should act more loving.*

It may make sense to remind couples of the words of the wise Salvador Minuchin at the 1999 Erickson Conference that *"Every marriage is a mistake. Some people just cope with their mistakes better than others."*

"Infidelity Is Normal; Everybody Does It."

There are other beliefs that doom marriages in crisis, beliefs held by therapists, by writers of self help books, by marriage partners, and by the friends and relatives they confide in at times of marital uproar or disillusionment. These include the belief that *infidelity is normal and everybody does it.* The corollary of this is that marriage is abnormal and perhaps unhealthy.

Human beings are monogamous, like other group hunters such as wolves, and like other nest building species such as rodents and birds (chickens are the exception). Many of us humans, rodents, and birds struggle with monogamy and at times feel attracted to other creatures. While we are monogamous by nature, human beings are adaptable and can be trained instead for polygamy, promiscuity, or serial monogamy. We can be seduced and distracted from monogamy by intense sexual attractions or by guilty secrets. In our promiscuous world, we must either be raised for monogamy or trained for it, preferably both. Happily, we have a cerebral cortex which helps us manage our impulses.

Married people are healthier, wealthier, and wiser than unmarried people, and a helluva lot happier than single people and particularly than divorced people. And this is true whether they like their specific husband or wife or not.

IF SOMEONE IS BEING UNFAITHFUL

Infidelity is prevalent among people who come to therapy, though therapists may go out of their way to avoid recognizing it. While infidelity is announced as the event that brings couples to therapy about 25% of the time, an even larger number will reveal it in the course of the therapy (Glass & Wright, 1992). A lot of therapists avoid dealing with infidelity because they don't know how (Whisman, Dixon, & Johnson, 1997).

Here is our best advice on how to deal with a crisis of infidelity:

1. The infidel needs to stop the affair. Completely. This may hurt, at least for a while, but we promise the hurt won't last.
2. The infidel needs to take total responsibility for breaking the marriage.
3. Defensiveness ("it is not my fault") is absolutely verboten.
4. The infidel needs to tell the truth as often as necessary and in as much detail as their spouse needs. Secrets keep the marriage from achieving intimacy and healing.
5. It helps for the infidel to tell the truth compassionately. Bader and Pearson (2000) give this wonderfully wise advice and its even wiser corollary:
6. It helps keep the truth flowing if the betrayed spouse hears the truth compassionately. Both steps will help betrayed spouses' traumatic reactions from becoming crystallized and chronic.
7. It helps for the couple to embark on a new courtship and reestablish intimacy with each other, giving the courtship their full attention.
8. The infidel may need to stay on as short a leash as the betrayed spouse requires, in order to know the affair is over.
9. Whining over the consequences the infidel brought on him/herself is superfluous and irritating.
10. The cuckolded partner's continued anger (once it is clear and out in the open that the betrayed partner is angry) is not helpful, for

him or her, or for the repair of the relationship, but it is not up to the infidel to determine when enough is enough. Therapists can provide some structure for the anger, and ensure the anger doesn't present a threat to safety, but should not try to suppress or ignore it, nor should the infidel.

11. If this affair were one of a series, you may be treating a philanderer, who needs to reexamine his/her training and philosophy about marriage, sex, honesty and gender. The problem is not in the marriage, but in the infidel's relationship with gender and family traditions.

12. If this affair was unique and intensely romantic and something for which the infidel was willing to give up a marriage, children, and half of his or her kingdom, the infidel was undoubtedly crazy and perhaps depressed. This affair might be considered a suicide equivalent. Romantic infidels need to look at the crisis in life that led to such a drastic action at this time.

13. If this affair was wildly out of character and had the accidental quality of "just happening," the infidel may not be guarding his or her boundaries well and may need a keeper.

14. When infidels are stuck between marriage and affair, they might try telling the truth at home and lying to the affair partner. Generally people will cling to whoever shares their secrets (Wegner, Lane, & Dimitri, 1994). The infidel must realize that, however he or she might like to, one can't have both and until one gets all the way in the boat or all the way on the dock, one is in danger of falling in. Those who can't decide may be better off sticking with the marriage: the odds are a lot better.

15. While it is rarely helpful for the therapist to attack the affairee personally, people who are screwing around should be told "Keep in mind that Miss or Mr. Wonderful wants something desperately, but is not a social worker and does not have the best interests of you and your loved ones at heart. People who screw around with married people are not noted for their stability or generosity or sanity. Beware."

MYTHS THAT WRECK MARRIAGE

There are certain widely held beliefs in society that doom marriage. They must be challenged by therapists and by the rest of us.

1. *Marriage is magical.* If this is the right marriage it won't take any work.
2. *Marriage is about being in love.* If you're not in love right this moment, it's an emergency requiring human sacrifice. (The obsession with not being in-love is of course a depressive state, but it may seem to amateurs that the problem is in the marriage itself.)
3. *Affairs are not your fault if your mate fails to make your life a constant state of ecstatic wonder,* i.e., if he or she stonewalls, criticizes, complains, or shows contempt. What's more, affairs are not your fault because you are a child and your marriage partner is the grownup who is supposed to meet your every need.
4. *If your marriage does not make you happy, you will surely be miserable,* unless you make your getaway, which is much too lonely and scary to do alone. You need a confederate in running away.
5. *Marital sins are unforgivable and marital breaks irretrievable;* once broken the marriage can never hold the lives it must hold. (The truth is that marriages can be far stronger after the successful resolution of a crisis of infidelity. Most growth is the outgrowth of crisis. It is a commonplace that "love fades." But as Rob Reiner said in *The Story of Us*, "Hate fades" too.)
6. *If you divide the tasks by gender, then there'll be less conflict and all will be well.* Men may believe if there is one designated captain of the ship then there can be no mutiny. Women may believe that men are such amateur human beings they should just consider themselves children and recognize that only females can be grownups. Many marriage counselors, perhaps coming from a background in religion rather than mental health, are uncomfortable with marital conflict and are willing to sacrifice the necessary conflict of negotiation and the building of intimacy in order to protect couples from fighting. The result might be efficient but impersonal, silent marriages.
7. *"The kids will be fine"* if the parents break up the family. While adults are too fragile to get along without getting their heart's desire, children are infinitely resilient and don't need parents at all. The data on children of divorce is appalling even as we try to normalize the painful procedure. Sure there are marriages that are a threat to life, limb, or sanity, and we strongly believe that given a choice between suicide, homicide, or divorce, divorce is preferable. Even then it is a disaster for children and parental remarriage is likely to be even more disastrous. Maybe one of the parents, or

rarely both of them, will be happier after a divorce, but the children are not likely to be since the marriages that end in divorce are unfortunately not the ones that are violent and crazy making and unsafe, but those in which someone is messing around looking for the fulfillment of some narcissistic fantasy of ideal love.

SKILLS FOR MONOGAMY

Monogamy may not come naturally, particular for children of divorce, those who have spent too long playing courtship games, or those who have already failed at a marriage or two and no longer trust the institution. But the skills for monogamy can be taught and the treatment of crises of infidelity involves teaching these skills. People who would be monogamous need to learn to:

1. *Aspire to equality*: you either both win or you both lose.
2. *Practice honesty* (telling the bad news first, showing the warts, stopping the gender dance and the pretence of heroism or perfection).
3. *Risk intimacy* ("knowing" requires hanging out together until you know each other so well you see life through binocular visions).
4. *Make the commitment* (*Get all the way in your marriage.*) Don't even ask yourself whether this is the right marriage. Ask instead whether you are doing the marriage right.
5. *Take on the identity of marriage* (It is who you are; divorce is out of the question, in the category of putting the kids up for adoption or moving to another planet.)
6. *Bolster your marriage*: Choose monogamous friends, people who support marriage in general and your marriage in particular.
7. *Keep it private*: Don't confide your marital complaints to amateurs. They can panic and try to protect you from your own marriage.
8. *Expand the emotional range*: Get yourself and your partner comfortable with the ups and downs of marriage.
9. *Hang in there.* Refuse to step back and fight distance with more distance.
10. Invest in the idea that *satisfaction with marriage is mostly your doing*.

11. Manners. *If all else fails try manners*. Maybe even kindness, politeness, and humility.

PROBLEMS FOR AMATEUR MONOGAMISTS

Some people have more trouble with marriage than others. Among those who have the hardest time with it are those:

1. People whose parents couldn't do marriage. Children of divorce have a painfully high divorce rate. They can still make marriage work but they will have to understand their parents' marriages and learn what their parents didn't know.
2. People whose parents could do marriage but felt put upon by it and, by complaining about it too much, poisoned the well.
3. People whose personal shame precludes letting themselves be known.
4. People who have ideals of inequality and are so afraid of losing the power struggle they try to win at marriage. *One can't be right and married at the same time.*
5. People who are influenced by societal anti-marriage messages which encourage you to protect yourself from it by keeping part of yourself out of it.
6. People who go to anti-marriage therapists, whether those therapists are feminist, masculinist, fundamentalist, paranoid, or just depressed and "unlucky" at love but nonetheless who reassure them that whatever they are doing is not their fault.
7. People who stereotype other people on the basis of gender. Any generalization anyone believes about gender is depersonalizing and dangerous in marriage.
8. People who didn't see their parents navigate conflict successfully may be left fearing marital conflict as a deal breaker rather than the business of the marriage.

THERAPISTS AND CRISIS OF INFIDELITY

Crises of infidelity require the help of a therapist. Like brain surgery, you shouldn't try it at home by yourself. All therapists, however, are not equally competent in dealing with crises of infidelity. To be successful with such cases, therapists must:

1. Believe in marriage.
2. See the benefits of marriage for kids and adults.
3. Seek character building opportunities in crisis.
4. Be unafraid of conflict but not in love with anger either.
5. Know and accept the life cycle of marriage.
6. Never compare anything as complex, rich and total as marriage, which abounds in reality, to something as shallow, two dimensional and ephemeral as an affair. Affairs are fantasies for people who are afraid to grow up; don't take them seriously.
7. Take infidelity very seriously. Post-traumatic reactions, in both partners, are frequent and can become chronic. Therapists must have the courage to safely and persistently explore the impact of the affair.

MARRIAGE WRECKING THERAPISTS

Some therapists are disastrous with infidelity crises. Those include:

1. Rescuers, either those who protect the victim from the villain or those who protect the perpetrator from guilt. Crises can be opportunities for many things, certainly for intimacy. Guilt ("I could have done better.") is good for you. It is shame ("I am weak and helpless and I can't help doing what I do") that disempowers and paralyzes.
2. Avenging angels who use their positions as therapists to punish imperfect mates.
3. Neutrals, who by not taking a stand, leave people's lives at the mercy of their feelings, in the throes of a crisis in which their feelings are utterly unreliable for reasons best explained by Helen Fisher (1992): the brain goes kaflooey when the boundaries are breached and the feelings are increasingly unreliable and disconnected from the realities of past, present and future.
4. Anti-marriage self-actualizers ("You deserve better.")
5. Romantics, who think marriages should conform to the therapist's fantasies.

AND FINALLY–

We believe all marriages are inherently incompatible. That gives them much of their energy as people go through life developing the binocular vision that comes from seeing every incident in life through both the lenses of your own experience and training and emotional responses and those of your partner. Each partner will surely have a different and enlightening set of lenses through which to see life. We have not believed one needs to marry the right person, but that one needs to <u>be</u> the right person. However, it is wise not just to believe in marital fidelity but to marry someone who also believes in marriage and monogamy.

The last word on this matter is simply that marriages can survive infidelity but they may not survive bad therapy.

REFERENCES

Amato, P., & Rogers, S. (1997). A longitudinal study of marital problems and subsequent divorce. *Journal of Marriage & the Family*, 59(3), 612-624.

Bader, E., & Pearson, P. (2000). *Tell me no lies.* NY: St. Martin's Press.

Fisher, H. (1992). *Anatomy of love.* NY: Norton.

Gilligan, C. (1982). *In a different voice.* Cambridge: Harvard University Press.

Glass, S. (2003). *Not "just friends."* NY: Simon and Schuster.

Glass, S.P. (1981). Sex differences in the relationship between satisfaction with various aspects of marriage and types of extramarital involvements (doctoral dissertation, Catholic University, 1980). *Dissertation Abstracts International*, 41(10), 3889B.

Glass, S.P., & Wright, T.L. (1992) Justifications for extramarital involvement: The association between attitudes, behavior, and gender. *Journal of Sex Research*, 29(3), 361-387.

Glass, S.P., & Wright, T.L. (1997). Reconstructing marriages after the trauma of infidelity. In W.K. Halford & H.J. Markman (Eds.), *Clinical Handbook of Marriage and Couples Intervention* (pp. 471-507) Chichester: Wiley.

Hunt, M. (1969). *The affair.* NY: World Publishing Company.

Jacobson, N., Dobson, K., Fruzzetti, A.E., Schmaling, K.B., & Salusky, S. (1991). Marital therapy as a treatment for depression. *Journal of Consulting and Clinical Psychology*, 59, 547-557.

Michael, R.T, Gagnon, J.H., Laumann, E.O., & Kolata, G. (1994). *Sex in America.* Boston: Little Brown.

Pittman, F., & Wagers, T. P. (1995). Crises of infidelity. In N. Jacobson & A. Gurman (Eds.) *Handbook of Couple Therapy.* NY: Guilford.

Pittman, F. (1987). *Turning points: Treating families in transition and crisis.* NY: Norton.

Pittman, F. (1989). *Private lies: Infidelity and the betrayal of intimacy.* NY: Norton.

Pittman, F. (1993). *Man enough: Fathers, sons, and the search for masculinity.* NY: Putnam.

Pittman, F. (1998). *Grow up! How taking responsibility can make you a happy adult.* NY: St. Martin's.

Rasmussen, P.K., & Ferraro, K.J. (1979). The divorce process. *Alternative Lifestyles* 2, 443-460.

Spanier,G., & Margolis,R. (1983). Marital separation and extramarital sexual behavior. *Journal of Sex Research,* 19(1), 23-48.

Treas, J., & Giesen, D. (2000). Sexual infidelity among married and cohabiting Americans. *Journal of Marriage and the Family*, 62(1), 48-60.

Wagers, T. P. (2003). Assessment of infidelity. In K. Jordan (Ed.), *Handbook of couple and family assessment*. Nova Science Publishers, 2003.

Wegner, D., Lane, J., & Dimitri, S. (1994). The allure of secret relationships. *Journal of Personality and Social Psychology*, 66(2), 287-300.

Whisman, M.A., Dixon, A.E., & Johnson, B. (1997). Therapists' perspectives of couple problems and treatment issues in the practice of couple therapy. *Journal of Family Psychology*, 11(3), 361-366.

A Family Systems Approach
to Working with Sexually Open
Gay Male Couples

Michael Bettinger

SUMMARY. The majority of gay male couples are not monogamous. Relationship clinicians can help gay male couples to have a healthy sexually open relationship by working from a family systems perspective. This approach requires the therapist to have an understanding of family systems theory, the Enneagram (a personality topology), gay male sexual culture, as well as being clear of negative countertransference. Assessment of functionality of sexually open gay male relationships is described. *[Article copies available for a fee from The Haworth Document Delivery Service: 1-800-HAWORTH. E-mail address: <docdelivery@haworthpress.com> Website: <http://www.HaworthPress.com> © 2005 by The Haworth Press, Inc. All rights reserved.]*

KEYWORDS. Homosexuality, sexuality, sexually open relationship, monogamy, polyamory, gay, couples, family systems, growth model, Enneagram

---

Dr. Michael Bettinger is a psychotherapist, educator, and writer. He is in private practice in San Francisco and works primarily with people who are gay, lesbian, bisexual, or transgendered.

[Haworth co-indexing entry note]: "A Family Systems Approach to Working with Sexually Open Gay Male Couples." Bettinger, Michael. Co-published simultaneously in *Journal of Couple & Relationship Therapy* (The Haworth Press) Vol. 4, No. 2/3, 2005, pp. 149-160; and: *Handbook of the Clinical Treatment of Infidelity* (ed: Fred P. Piercy, Katherine M. Hertlein, and Joseph L. Wetchler) The Haworth Press, Inc., 2005, pp. 149-160. Single or multiple copies of this article are available for a fee from The Haworth Document Delivery Service [1-800-HAWORTH, 9:00 a.m. - 5:00 p.m. (EST). E-mail address: docdelivery@haworthpress.com].

Same-sex couples are no longer an oddity to most people. Same-sex marriage is now legal in a number of countries and is being debated in America. It appears increasingly likely that same-sex couples will request the services of skilled relationship clinicians to help develop more functional relationships. Many of these gay male couples will not be monogamous.

Effective work with gay male couples require clinicians to have skills that are both similar to and different from the skills needed when working with opposite-sex couples. The similar skills include a basic understanding of family systems theory and its therapeutic applications as well as being fairly free of negative countertransference regarding human sexuality. The different skills include clinicians having knowledge of, and a non-judgmental attitude toward the culture of gay male sexuality, and an understanding of the particular dynamics that can lead to problems in a sexually open relationship. All of these skills can be learned. This paper will discuss these skills and describe a family systems approach to facilitate working with gay male couples who have a sexually open relationship and who wish to discuss the nature of their sexuality while working with a relationship clinician.

GAY MALE SEXUAL CULTURE AND OPEN RELATIONSHIPS

Understanding the following aspects of the culture of gay male sexuality should help a relationship clinician to work more effectively with gay male couples. The majority of gay male couples are not monogamous, and the longer a gay male couple is together, the less likely they are to have a monogamous relationship (Bell & Weinberg, 1978; Blumstein & Schwartz, 1983; McWhirter & Mattison, 1984; Saghir & Robins, 1973). While there appears to be a bias toward monogamy in the general culture, within the gay male culture the bias appears to be toward sexually open relationships.

In mainstream society, monogamy, and sexually open relationships are frequently framed in moral terms. Those in monogamous relationships are often described as being committed, dedicated, devoted, faithful, loyal, and reliable. A non-monogamous married person is often described as deceitful, dishonest, disloyal, false, two-faced, or unfaithful. He or she is described as having engaged in adultery, betrayal, cheating, cuckoldry, debauchery, duplicity, faithlessness, falseness, fornication, immorality, infidelity, perfidy, promiscuity, sin, or treachery. Mainstream society has historically condemned sexual contact outside of marriage.

In the American gay male community, monogamy is generally approached as a morally neutral issue, and dealt with in practical, not moral terms. The prevailing question for many gay male couples is not whether monogamy is good or bad, or right or wrong, but whether monogamy would help or hurt the couple. Most gay male couples decide it is not in their interest to be monogamous. Should this be their decision, a relationship clinician can help to make that decision work better for them.

Within the American gay male culture, there is also acceptance and support for anonymous sexual encounters. In every city and town in America, there are cruising areas where men can go to meet other men for brief sexual encounters. Gay travel guide books always list these areas. As the size of the towns and cities increase, the number of commercial establishments that cater to this desire, such as bars, bathhouses, sex clubs, adult bookstores, and movie houses, increases. The Internet has added a new and powerful means for men to connect with other men for sexual activity. Within the gay male community, overwhelmingly the existence of these establishments and practices are discussed in morally neutral terms.

Some gay men practice polyamory (Bettinger, in press), which can also be understood as a form of responsible non-monogamy. These men have more than one ongoing sexual relationships that are stable, committed and endure over time. The intricacies of these relationships can be complex. Within the gay male community, polyamorous relationships are also generally discussed in morally neutral terms.

Mainstream society subtly encourages everyone, including gay men, to focus on the sexual aspect of who gay men are. Gay men and gay male couples are labeled and defined by mainstream society by the nature of their sexuality to a much greater extent than is true for heterosexual individuals or couples. Frequently the term gay is added as a descriptor when talking about an individual or couple who happens to be attracted to members of their own sex, whether or not the issue being discussed is related to sexual behavior. Thus gay men are subtly and frequently directed to focus on the part of their nature that relates to sexual activity.

Additionally, gay male couples are composed only of men. All men, from the time they are young, are exposed to a multitude of messages encouraging them to be sexual. It should not, therefore, be surprising that sexuality is an important and ever present issue for gay men and gay male couples. All this results in a subculture of sexuality within the gay male community that is significantly different from the mainstream culture of sexuality, and understanding that culture helps a relationship clinician to work effectively with gay male couples.

WORKING ON COUNTERTRANSFERENCE

When working with gay male couples who have sexually open relationships, clinicians are exposed to three highly charged emotional subjects; sexuality, homosexuality, and sexually open relationships. These subjects are likely to produce some countertransference in all relationship clinicians. Countertransference is the conscious and unconscious process resulting in the clinician experiencing positive, negative, and/or neutral feelings in response to clients (Slakter, 1987).

The previous frank discussion of the gay male sexual culture is likely to have brought up feelings in the reader. The following section should help the reader to understand more about his or her reaction. It should give some insight to what he or she believes about human sexuality and where some of those beliefs come from. This author encourages all relationship clinicians to understand and accept that he or she has a particular set of beliefs about human sexuality that can be described, discussed, thought about, and sometimes changed. To the extent they are negative they can have a negative impact on one's clinical work. I believe it is impossible for anyone, including all relationship clinicians, to grow up and live in this society without internalizing certain negative messages regarding human sexuality, homosexuality, and sexually open relationships.

Models of Sexual Behavior

A relationship clinician can be more aware of his or her countertransference by understanding the model(s) of human behavior, particularly regarding human sexuality, to which he or she subscribes. A "model" of human behavior is a set of general principles held by the clinician that explains why people behave as they do. It enables someone to organize disparate facts into a cohesive understanding of human behavior (Bettinger, 2001). There are four models of human behavior that are relevant here, the supernatural model, the moral model, the medical model, and the growth model. To some degree, each of us holds beliefs based in all four of these models and the combinations result in each clinician having a unique way of understanding human behavior and human sexuality. This is also true for our clients.

To the extent that a clinician holds beliefs regarding sexual behavior that are based in the supernatural, moral, or the medical model, he or she will have to some degree have a negative countertransference. The growth model is the one least likely to result in a negative countertransference. Understanding the nature of the supernatural, moral, and medical models regarding sexuality can help a clinician to identify within him or herself some aspects of negative countertransference and to take whatever actions are possible and appropriate.

The Supernatural Model. The supernatural model suggests that God, Satan, spirits, demons, or other supernatural forces can take over an individual and control his or her behavior. While few clinicians can acknowledge without embarrassment that they hold beliefs based in the supernatural model regarding human sexuality, I find many actually do. Western religions and popular culture reinforce connecting the devil or demons to sexual acts. My clients (some of whom have been mental health clinicians) have acknowledged to me that at times they have had highly erotic and enjoyable sexual fantasies with demonic or satanic themes. Some are general and undefined, such as their sexuality having something to do with aspects of the "dark" side. Other fantasies are more specific, such as being "possessed" by a demonic force, or forced to be sexual with a demonic creature. In the same vein, sermons given by priests and ministers regularly refer to Satan's attempts to control humans, including through sexual behaviors. We are all regularly exposed to this kind of thinking. To the extent that clinicians have internalized some of these views, even if only on a deep level, will cause them to view sexuality in a negative way.

The Moral Model. The moral model is perhaps the most problematic. It permeates many aspects of our society. It suggests there is an intellectually and religiously determined correct way to behave. It postulates that an individual has free will and chooses to act in either good or evil ways, and can change from acting in an evil way to acting in a good way.

The problem is the moral model is based on an arbitrary set of assumptions that is not universally agreed upon. While some aspects of the moral model have almost universal acceptance, such as that murder is wrong, many of the sexual and pleasure oriented behaviors that the moral model condemns have widespread practice and acceptance by a minority of the population. Until recently the moral model has held that homosexuality and sex outside of a committed relationship are morally wrong. The morality of homosexuality is now being extensively debated. By comparison, there is almost no debate regarding the frequently stated belief that sex outside a relationship is morally wrong. Beliefs that consensual adult sexual behavior can be arbitrarily classified as either good or bad, right or wrong, based on moral and religious opinions will result in a negative countertransference.

The Medical Model. The medical model suggests that certain behaviors be seen as indicative of mental illness. The medical model is also problematic for several reasons. First, it appears to have influenced by the moral model concerning sexuality. Second, it attempts to see sexual behavior as either evidence, or the lack thereof, of a mental disease process. While some aspects of human behavior clearly has organic roots, most aspects of human behavior is much more complex. Those believing in a medical model have now backtracked from their formerly and firmly held belief that homosexuality is a mental illness. But other aspects of human sexual behavior, such as sexual fetishes, paraphilias, and consensual sadomasochism are still sometimes considered to be indicative of mental illness (American Psychiatric Association, 1994). The medical model is the dominant model regarding mental health in America, and most psychotherapeutic theoretical orientations are based in the medical model.

The Growth Model. The growth model suggests behavior be seen as an individual doing what he or she believes is needed to continue to grow as a functional person. The basic assumption of the growth model is that people have a desire and a need to grow over the course of their lives, they want to do it "right." To be emotionally healthy, a person must believe he or she is growing in ways that fit him or her. Symptoms of emotional distress appear when growth is inhibited. Obstacles to growth are present in distorted ideas learned earlier in life or in interactions with others in the present.

The growth model removes sexual behavior from the realm of the supernatural, the moral or the medical, and places it on a pragmatic level where the impact can be objectively discussed. The clinician's job is to help clients understand their innermost motives, help them assess their own level of functioning, and analyze where the origins of their difficulties to assist them to grow in healthy ways

The more clinicians understand their own unique views on human sexuality, the more they are able to understand how their views might impact their clinical work surrounding these highly charged emotional issues. The clearer and less judgmental relationship clinicians become regarding sexuality, homosexuality and sexually open relationships, the more meaningful the issues discussed will be for their clients.

A FAMILY SYSTEMS APPROACH
TO SEXUALLY OPEN RELATIONSHIPS

The following approach to relationship counseling with gay male couples who have sexually open relationships enables the clinician to understand the story of the clients sexuality and the clients to discuss their sexuality as appropriate. This approach is based on two concepts which are even more specific models of human behavior. Both are based in the growth model. The first is family systems theory and its therapeutic applications (Fogarty, 1976; Guerin, 1978; Gurman & Kniskern, 1981; Leveton, 1984). Family systems theory helps us to understand the impact of the past, including the role(s) assigned a person in his family of origin. Family systems theory also helps us to understand how the systemic forces in the present makes change easy or difficult. The second is the Enneagram (Palmer, 1995; Riso & Hudson, 1999), a personality topology. This helps clients and clinicians understand what clients are attempting to achieve in this world through their sexual behavior. The Enneagram also identifies likely interactional patterns between individuals, and such information is helpful when combined with family systems theory in trying to understand what is going on in a relationship.

The approach begins by asking the relationship clinician to look at sexual behavior not in isolation but in a context. Sex, in or out of a relationship, is never "just sex." Sex is part of a person's entire romantic, emotional, and sexual mating pattern; how he goes about connecting and being intimate with others. It is also for many a spiritual experience. This approach also assumes people have some control over their mating patterns and that they are making choices. This enables clinicians to help clients look at the probable consequences of their behavioral choices. Behaviors say much about what a person desires sexually.

A number of concepts from family systems theory are relevant when trying to work with sexually open gay male couples. Family systems theory believes that relationships are homeostatic systems (Leveton, 1984; Luthman, 1974). Homeostasis is the mechanism by which a family or relationship maintains the status quo by balancing various needs and behaviors in such a way that small risks in the name of growth can be tolerated. From this perspective, sexual activity outside the relationship can either stabilize the relationship and preserve the homeostasis, or it can destabilize the relationship. It should not be assumed that sex outside a relationship necessarily destabilizes a relationship. Such assumptions are often based in the moral model.

The family systems approach also includes a theory of positive intent (Luthman, 1974). Positive intent means that people want to grow, and their behavior reflects this desire. They are forever trying to do better. Sexual behavior becomes one of many morally neutral subjects. The question is whether the particular sexual behavior is consistent with growth and being a higher functioning person, or are the behaviors ultimately self defeating for this purpose. Either is possible.

The theory of positive intent postulates that all sex outside the relationship, whether it appears to be functional or dysfunctional, is an attempt by the client to help himself and his partner to grow as human beings. It is designed to improve, not destroy. Whether it is successful needs to be assessed. Understanding the specific nature of the positive intent often leads to a clearer understanding of why a particular sexual activity is going on.

Family systems theory believes that each family or relationship has a complex set of rules and roles which are understood and accepted on both an explicit and implicit level by the family members. The function of these rules and roles is to permit the family to survive in the greater society (Leveton, 1984; Luthman, 1974; Satir, 1972, 1983). We learn these rules and roles in our family of origin, and find partners with whom we attempt to continue to act out these rules and roles in our adulthood. Sexual behavior, both within and outside one's primary partner occurs within the context of these rules and roles.

Empirical research has not yet been done to understand what roles that children who will grow up to be gay men most often get assigned in their family of origin. Some of the more common roles assigned to children are that of the good child, the happy child, the family hero, the problem child, the lost child, the scapegoat, the bad child, the rebel, the "different" child, and the sexual child. My experience has been that gay children somehow more often gets assigned the negative roles disproportionate to their frequency in the family. The positive intent for the family is that this enables at least one family member to express something that needs expression, but is otherwise unexpressed or unexpressible in the family, particularly as it relates to sexuality. These roles remain in the adult identity of the gay man.

It is the rebel, the different one, the sexual one, along with the good child, the family hero, etc., that is being sexual outside a relationship as an adult. Individual needs related to those roles also get met by the sexual activity. These include non-sexual needs, such as a need for excitement, adventure, danger, intensity, pleasure, validation, love, independence, creative self expression, conquest, or achievement. Yet another person may be seeking to create a wider support network through meeting people in a sexual context. Family systems theory helps us to understand that sexual activity occurs in a complex context and understanding that context helps us to discuss the sexual activity in a more rational and less judgmental manner.

THE ENNEAGRAM

The Enneagram, a growth model based on personality topology, further helps us to understand what an individual is trying to achieve in life through all behavior, including sexual activity. The Enneagram postulates that there are nine personality types, and many subtypes. It uses terminology that non-mental health professionals can understand. Within each personality type is a discussion of that type's greatest hopes, worst fears, essential needs, among others. Clients can usually accurately determine their type. One of the greatest benefits of the Enneagram is that it jump starts a client's vocabulary to describe who he is and what he is about. It enables him to communicate to, or to understand his partner, regarding sexual activity in a personal and contextual way. Through the knowledge of the self that a person gains from understanding his Enneagram type, he is more able to personally own what are the great themes in his life and communicate them to his partner in a way his partner can understand. The result is usually each member of the couple being able to understand and accept themselves and their partner on a broader level.

While different writers use slightly different terms to label the various personality types, all are similar, emphasizing subtle nuances of each personality type. I believe the best overall description of the Enneagram is by Riso and Hudson (1999). Palmer (1995) describes the likely interactional patterns between the Enneagram personality types when those individuals either work together or are in an intimate relationship. Together with the family role of each individual, the sexual behavior can be discussed in a personal and meaningful relational context.

ASSESSMENT OF FUNCTIONALITY IN SEXUALLY OPEN GAY MALE RELATIONSHIPS

How well or poorly a gay male couple does regarding their open relationship can be assessed by looking at a number of dynamics that pertain to their open relationship. Assessment of these dynamics by the clinician and/or the couple can indicate to either where work is necessary. It should be noted that these dynamics are present in all relationships, and they are not the only dynamics that are important to assess regarding couples who have sexually open relationships. But these dynamics do have special meaning regarding sexually open relationships.

Honesty

The essential question here is how honest is each partner regarding his sexual behavior. Lack of honesty regarding sexual behavior is perhaps the dynamic that leads to the most trouble. Sexuality is a highly charged emotional issue. While all couples need honesty, the possibilities for triangulation and chaos increase when couples are having sexually open relationships. It is important to note that honesty does not mean telling one's partner everything. That is a boundary issue that each gay male couple must decide; how much is to be shared, how much is to be kept private, and what is to be kept secret. It is being honest about whether one is following through on what has been previously agreed upon that is important.

Jealousy, Envy, and Possessiveness

The essential question here is to what level is either partner experiencing jealousy, envy and/or possessiveness, and how are those emotions being handled? These emotions exist in everyone. They are natural and normal, and often serve functional purposes. However, when a gay male couple has a sexually open relationship, it is necessary to sexually share one's partner with others. This almost inevitably brings up some feelings of jealousy, envy, and possessiveness. The couple can use the therapy hour to learn to be less jealous, envious and possessive. Each partner is capable of learning to respect the other relationships their partner is having. Doing that increases the functionality of the couple.

Boundaries

The essential questions here are how clear are the boundaries and how well are they respected. Having a sexually open relationship does not usually mean either partner can do whatever he wants, whenever he wants. Relationships become more functional when the couple agrees on the "who," "what," "where," "when," and "how" issues regarding sexual behavior. Some typical boundary issues in sexually open gay male relationships are as follows. When is someone expected to be with their primary partner, and when can they be with others? What sexual acts are permitted outside the relationship and which are not? Is anything excluded? For instance, an HIV-negative couple might decide to exclude anal intercourse with others, as unprotected receptive anal intercourse is the primary means by which HIV is transmitted within the gay male community. Is it OK to bring someone to the home shared by both, or must the sexual activity take place in other locations? Clarity and follow through of the boundary issues should be assessed.

Health and Safe Sex Issues

The essential question here is to what degree is either partner putting his own or others' health at risk. With an increasing number of partners, a gay man risks exposure to a number of sexually transmitted diseases, including HIV and hepatitis C, both of which are widespread in the gay community and can be life threatening. To the extent that a gay man is or is not protecting himself or others from exposure to sexually transmitted diseases, it is indicative of his level of functioning, and is another area to be assessed.

AREA FOR FUTURE RESEARCH

Gay male couples are as well functioning and satisfied with their relationship as are married heterosexual couples, and score significantly higher on those scales than do divorced heterosexual couples (Green, Bettinger, & Zacks, 1996). An area for future research would be to see if there is any difference in relationship satisfaction between gay male couples who are monogamous and those who have sexually open relationships.

CONCLUSION

Many gay male couples have sexually open relationships and it is more likely than ever that these couples will seek the help of relationship clinicians to improve their relationships. Relationship clinicians can improve the work they do with these couples by understanding and accepting the culture of gay male sexuality, ridding themselves of negative countertransference to the extent possible, and using a family systems approach when working with them.

REFERENCES

American Psychiatric Association. (1994). *Diagnostic and statistical manual of mental disorders: Fourth edition.* Washington, DC: American Psychiatric Association.

Bell, A., & Weinberg, M. (1978). *Homosexualities: A study of diversities among men and women.* New York: Simon and Schuster.

Bettinger, M. (in press). Polyamory and gay men: A family systems approach. *Journal of GLBT Family Studies.*

Bettinger, M. (2001). *It's your hour: A guide to queer affirmative psychotherapy.* Los Angeles: Alyson.

Blumstein, P., & Schwartz, P. (1983). *American couples: Money, work, and sex.* New York: William Morrow & Company.

Fogarty, T. F. (1976). Systems concepts and the dimensions of self. In Guerin, P. J. (Ed.), *Family Therapy.* (pp. 144-153). New York: Gardner Press.

Green, R-J., Bettinger, M., & Zacks, E. (1996). Are lesbian couples fused and gay male couples disengaged?: Questioning gender straightjackets. In J. Laird & R-J. Green (Eds.), *Lesbians and gays in couples and families: A handbook for therapists* (pp. 185-230). San Francisco: Jossey-Bass.

Guerin, P.J. (1978). *Family therapy: Theory and practice.* New York: Gardner Press.

Gurman, A.S., & Kniskern, D.P. (Eds.). (1981). *Handbook of family therapy: Volume 1* New York: Brunner/Mazel.

Leveton, E. (1984). *Adolescent crisis: Family counseling approaches.* New York: Springer Publishing Company.

Luthman, S. G. (1974). *The dynamic family.* Palo Alto, CA: Science and Behavior Books, Inc.

McWhirter, D., & Mattison, A. (1984). *The male couple.* Englewood Cliffs, NJ: Prentice-Hall.

Palmer, H. (1995). *The Enneagram in love and work: Understanding your intimate and business relationships.* New York: Harper Collins.

Riso, D., & Hudson, H. (1999). *The wisdom of the Enneagram: The complete guide to the psychological and spiritual growth for the nine personality types.* New York: Bantaan Books.

Saghir, M., & Robins, E. (1973). *Male and female homosexuality: A Comprehensive Investigation.* Baltimore, MD: Williams and Wilkins.

Satir, V. (1972). *Peoplemaking.* Palo Alto, CA: Science and Behavior Books.

Satir, V. (1983). *Conjoint family therapy.* (3rd ed.). Palo Alto, CA: Science and Behavior Books.

Slakter, E. (Ed.). (1987). *Countertransference: A comprehensive view of those reactions of the therapist to the patient that may help or hinder treatment.* New York: Jason Aronson Press.

Your Cheatin' Heart:
Myths and Absurdities
About Extradyadic Relationships

Scott Johnson

SUMMARY. This work challenges therapists to look at themselves and their beliefs regarding affairs. The work also examines common illogical beliefs in regards to extradyadic involvement. The reader is challenged to examine the underlying dynamic of extradyadic relationships and how their own biases affect how they view clients and work with the dyad. *[Article copies available for a fee from The Haworth Document Delivery Service: 1-800-HAWORTH. E-mail address: <docdelivery@haworthpress.com> Website: <http://www.HaworthPress.com> © 2005 by The Haworth Press, Inc. All rights reserved.]*

KEYWORDS. Extradyadic relationships, infidelity, affairs

Few topics are more riddled with mythical nonsense than the subject of extradyadic–meaning "outside of the couple"–relationships, and that is understandable. Few of us think rationally about things we often label uncontrollable, like sexual and emotional impulses.

Scott Johnson, PhD, is Associate Professor and Director, Marriage and Family Therapy Doctoral Program, Virginia Tech, Blacksburg, VA 24061-0515.

[Haworth co-indexing entry note]: "Your Cheatin' Heart: Myths and Absurdities About Extradyadic Relationships." Johnson, Scott. Co-published simultaneously in *Journal of Couple & Relationship Therapy* (The Haworth Press) Vol. 4, No. 2/3, 2005, pp. 161-172; and: *Handbook of the Clinical Treatment of Infidelity* (ed: Fred P. Piercy, Katherine M. Hertlein, and Joseph L. Wetchler) The Haworth Press, Inc., 2005, pp. 161-172. Single or multiple copies of this article are available for a fee from The Haworth Document Delivery Service [1-800-HAWORTH, 9:00 a.m. - 5:00 p.m. (EST). E-mail address: docdelivery@ haworthpress.com].

But thinking carefully about extradyadic relationships is critical. Few days go by in American life or elsewhere on the globe where someone, frequently a woman, is not killed for what the legal system still labels "adultery," that puzzling term used in the Old Testament, or what is often called, whether applied to married or unmarried partners, "cheating." Often such murders are accompanied by suicides and other killings, and children are frequently left orphaned or wards of the state, through the actions of people habituated to thinking of extradyadic relationships as worthy of both vigilante justice and capital punishment at a stroke. Occasionally, the children of the couple themselves are butchered, a response to extradyadic involvements as old as Medea.

Arguably, scholars and therapists often unwittingly encourage such behavior by carelessly adopting clearly judgmental terms for extradyadic behavior–the term "infidelity" is a common example–or by exaggerating the sense of victimization that extradyadic relationships entail. While there is no question extradyadic relationships can be a painful, shame filled experience for everyone they touch, there is also little question that they are often far more complex than simple, Frankie and Johnny, "he done her wrong" characterizations usually imply.

As scholars, we want to believe our pronouncements on extradyadic unions– or simply "affairs," as they are colloquially and relatively neutrally called–are at least logically consistent, if not ultimately provable or true. Yet a close examination of several common scholarly ideas about extradyadic involvements, such as their relative prevalence among men and women, or the presumed differing attractions of affairs for women and men, or even an affair's fundamental purpose in the context of a given relationship, including the question of who is victimizing whom, suggest many accepted theories are riddled with holes.

WHO'S CHEATIN' WHO

One of the most common illogical beliefs about affairs, for example, is that because surveys show men as a group reporting more extradyadic involvement than women, individual men must engage in affairs more frequently than individual women, an idea whose mathematical impossibility should be fairly obvious.

If there are roughly equal numbers of males and females in the population, for example, as nearly all censuses have told us, and if men as a group tend to have more heterosexual affairs than women tend to have, then *individual* men who have affairs must have *fewer* involvements than individual women who have affairs, if our calculations mean anything. Yet this is hardly ever what anyone concludes.

It may be easier to understand this if we forget, for the moment, affairs entirely and think about a totally different but equally heterosexual activity–mixed doubles tennis. Let's try out, for example, the assertion that we have made about affairs on mixed doubles tennis: "More men play mixed doubles tennis than women." Now, unless our mathematical skills have abandoned us entirely, the first question that should come to mind for us is: how in the world is that possible? For mixed doubles tennis by definition requires one man and one woman per side. How could more men play mixed doubles tennis than women?

There is of course only one possible answer, assuming our basic assertion is true: the individual men who play mixed doubles tennis must play *less frequently* than the individual women who play. (I have *absolutely* no idea if that is the case, by the way. This is a "hypothetical," as pollsters like to say.)

In turn, of course, that would mean those women who do engage in mixed doubles tennis must, on average, engage in it *more*–and not less–frequently than men. For if *equal* numbers of men and women played mixed doubles tennis, they both would have to play it about the same amount. But if *fewer* women played mixed doubles tennis than men, men would have to play mixed doubles *less frequently,* on average, than women.

All this can quickly get confusing, so let's augment our "hypothetical" with some numbers. Hypothetically, let's say, 22 men and 14 women play mixed doubles tennis in the course of a year. But for all of these men and women to each play at least once, the women would have to play nearly *twice* as frequently, on the whole, as the men. That is, the women who play would have to have "multiple partners" much more frequently than the men did, if all the men got to play at least once. Or just divide 22 by 14, and then try to divide 14 by 22, and decided which yields the larger number.

Okay, back to sex. And let's use the same numbers, since they come, in fact, from Greeley, Michael, and Smith's (1990) study of monogamy, in which 22% of sexually active men and 14% of sexually active women were found to be heterosexually "non-monogamous" (another less stigmatizing term that we might use). Given the fact that the proportions in the general population of women and men are within a percent or two of each other, the implication of their study is as obvious for affairs as it would be for mixed doubles tennis: women who are "non-monogamous" must be non-monogamous *much more frequently*–nearly *twice* as frequently, in fact–as non-monogamous men. Otherwise, the figures make no sense.

Yet this, of course, is totally contrary to what "we all know," is it not? We all know that men who have affairs have more affairs than women who get extradyadically involved, right? That's just the way men are, we say. Except men who have affairs *can't,* mathematically, have more frequent affairs than women who have affairs do; not if there are more men overall having affairs than women. Just as with mixed doubles tennis, if more men are playing in the first place than women, then the women who play with them *have to play more frequently* for all the men to get to play at all. The numbers simply won't work otherwise.

It's important for me to try to be clear here, because what I'm *not* trying to argue is that in fact there is any difference in the rate at which men and women have affairs in the first place (though most studies suggest–unconvincingly, in my book–there is). What I *am* saying is that if any of those studies–and there are dozens of them, ranging from Smith's (1991) finding that 2% of men and 1% of women have affairs to Hansen's (1987) claim that 71% of men versus 57% of women have extradyadic involvements–if *any* of them are true–and virtually all of them suggest that higher proportions of men have affairs than women–if *any* of that is accurate, then it can *only* mean that women who have affairs have them anywhere from roughly half again to twice as frequently as men who have affairs. Otherwise, all the numbers are *meshugeh.*

Either equal proportions of men and women are having affairs in the first place, in which case *nobody* is having more frequent affairs, relatively speaking, than anyone else, or whichever group is having a higher percentage of affairs has to have *fewer* affairs per individual than people in the other group.

Interestingly, mathematicians who follow such numbers occasionally try to point all this out to us. But we never seem to listen to them. The key, of course, is not to imagine we're talking about sex, which seems to get us all confused, but about tennis.

LOOKIN' FOR LOVE

Another of our shakier concepts concerning affairs has to do with the question of what men and women go into affairs searching for. Stereotypically–I'm trusting we don't need citations here–the thesis is that men engage in extradyadic relationships for sexual gratification and women for the "companionship." Sometimes this is expressed, as it often is by academic or clinical guests on radio or television talk shows, as affairs for men being about the "physical relationship" while for women they're about "intimacy."

But this view should raise several questions. For example, if it's true, then why don't men just masturbate, and why don't women just talk on the phone, or exchange love letters with their boyfriends? Or why don't men who have affairs simply have sex with their wives or regular partners, if sex is all they want? Why do men who have affairs fantasize about marrying their paramours, or stereotypically engage in conversations about feeling "misunderstood" by their partners, if "getting their rocks off" really is their only goal?

Are women who have affairs engaging in sex just as a kind of crude barter–"you give me talk and I'll give you sex?" Are men who offer flowers or love letters, romantic trips, dinners, presents, who tell their lovers "I couldn't wait to hear your voice," simply throwing out loss leaders to get their paramours into bed?

Or why, if it is just physical, do we then believe that men seek out multiple partners whereas women tend to have fewer paramours (which, as we noted above, could only mean *more* women overall are having affairs than men), since if you just want something physical, why change partners, if that's what you've already got? Wouldn't we expect women to want to have *more* partners since they could have more emotional involvements that way?

Looked at carefully, there seems little serious research which really supports this schizophrenic view of men and women's interest in extradyadic unions, and virtually all that we otherwise know about sexuality itself suggests it is a serious distortion.

Some of the problem, of course, may come from our confusing what people *seem to do* with what they actually *want*. In the recent film, *Something's Gotta Give*, for example, which featured Jack Nicholson as a purportedly sex obsessed record producer and Diane Keaton as an apparently willfully celibate playwright, one of the strongest messages is that what each *claims* to desire and even *seems* to desire is not in fact what they *actually* long for–a truth that shouldn't be hard for psychotherapists to digest.

The "womanizing" Nicholson character in fact becomes deeply emotionally attached to Keaton's aloof self-abnegater; Keaton's playwright becomes deeply lustful and sexually fulfilled. Wiser, perhaps, than us, the film seems to suggest not an *opposition* of sex and emotion, or some splitting of interest in them between men and women, but the obvious *harmony* between the physical and the affective–an idea we seem to embrace in nearly all other circumstances but are curiously reluctant to apply to extradyadic partners.

And yet, it was Masters and Johnson, after all, who showed us that sex is *not* "just physical," but as they often put it, a form of *communication.* What is the point of so much of the sex therapy we do, of the work of Horney and Kaplan and even Freud, if we really believe "sex" and "emotion" can truly be separated?

How could we work with the couples whom we see in sex therapy, if we really thought this was the case? Why would we encourage partners to talk about their sexual desires, their fantasies, their past experiences and levels of comfort; why come up with theories about attachment and its role in couples' lives if sex and emotion were somehow different things, or if women and men truly only wanted separate parts of the whole we otherwise see sex and emotion as?

After all, it wasn't the female country singer Reba McEntire, but the male vocalist Johnny Lee who came out with "Lookin' for Love (in all the wrong places)" in 1990. And while we might change the word "love" to "sex," suspecting the former is just a euphemism for the latter, the lines of the song tell a different story:

> I've spent a lifetime looking for you
> Single bars and good time lovers, never true
> Playing a fools game, hoping to win
> Telling those sweet lies and losing again.
>
> I was looking for love in all the wrong places
> Looking for love in too many faces
> Searching your eyes, looking for traces
> Of what . . . I'm dreaming of. . .
> Hopin' to find a friend and a lover
> God bless the day I discovered
> Another heart, lookin' for love. (Lee, 1990)

(Country music, by the way, *never* assumes more men than women "cheat." Garth Brooks, who sang the hit, "Papa Loved Mama" about a trucker who finds his wife in a motel with another man and rams his tractor-trailer through their room *["Mama's in the graveyard, Papa's in the pen"];* and Kenny Rogers, who sang about a wheelchair bound Vietnam Vet whose wife, "Ruby," regularly "took her love to town," both could testify to that.)

WHAT'S IT ALL ABOUT

And then we come to the problem of the underlying dynamic of extradyadic relationships–what, for individual couples, affairs are really "about." Too often, even serious researchers, seeking such answers, fall into the trap of seeing affairs largely as *moral* struggles with relational dimensions rather than *relational* struggles with moral dimensions, referring to the non-involved partner in a couple as the "betrayed," and the involved partner as the "infidel," rather than looking for systemic and psychological processes affecting both.

And general use of terms like "infidelity" or "betrayal" are in any case belied by a wealth of clinical experience, as well as theory. It was Carl Whitaker, after all, decades ago, who talked about the "mutual affair," in which, while the "infidel" of the couple might be physically and emotionally involved with another adult, the nominally "betrayed" partner could easily be "having an affair" with something or someone else–work, perhaps, or alcohol, or sports–do we not talk about football and golf "widows?" Or children, or organizations like school or church–do we not describe some people as "married" to church or children? Or families of origin–think of the many relationships where one partner remains fused with her or his childhood family. Or even to ideals–"duty," "honor," "respectability"? While certainly this is not always the case, it is often very hard for dispassionate observers to square such realities with any credible labels like "victim" and "betrayer."

Even the common idea of the secret nature of affairs is suspect, since many extradyadic relationships simply aren't. One thinks, for example, of the old joke about the paramour weeping helplessly at the funeral of his married lover, so inconsolable that the widowed husband comes over and puts his arm around him in genuine sympathy and says, "Do not worry, my friend. I will marry again."

And few of us, I would wager, imagine Hillary Clinton had been unaware of her presidential husband's philandering, yet it hardly takes great therapeutic insight to recognize that her secondary psychological gain, as we might term it, from her husband's behavior, like that of a large number of other political spouses, was quite vast.

While some of us wondered why she didn't simply dump him, even more people apparently saw her as a victim who nonetheless was "standing by her man," as Tammy Wynette put it so well many years ago. As commentators frequently noted, Bill Clinton's philandering actually humanized his wife to the public, melting what had seemed to be an aloofness and estrangement from traditional female roles. More than a few pundits, in fact, suggested her election to the Senate was not unrelated to the sympathy generated by her husband's dalliances, an office she conceivably might not have won without, among other advantages, the *bas relief of* Bill's Oval Office trysts.

And an even better example of the complex relational dynamics of affairs comes, as we might expect, from another political family, the Kennedys, whose family genogram was compiled by Randy Gersen and Monica McGoldrick (1985).

One of the fairly obvious things their family patterns show, for example, is that affairs among the Kennedy men aren't simply about relationships with their wives; and, far from being intended as "betrayals" of family trust, they are really intergenerational *homages* to their male ancestors, clear messages of loyalty and acceptance from sons to their fathers, or fathers-in-law.

Young Joe Kennedy, Sr., for example, seeking the hand of Rose Fitzgerald, the daughter of Boston's then-mayor, known as "Honey Fitz"–do we have to ask where he got the name?–could not have helped but notice that his future father-in-law was involved with a woman named "Toodles" Ryan, whose profession has come down to us as "cigarette girl." Subsequently, Joe Kennedy, Sr., had numerous affairs himself, including one with the Hollywood starlet, Gloria Swanson, in clear imitation of Honey Fitz himself. But his son Jack–who tellingly was named for his wandering maternal grandfather–undoubtedly went both of them several better, having many liaisons, and becoming involved not simply with a starlet like Swanson, but the greatest sex symbol of them all, Marilyn Monroe. Clearly, this was far less a pattern of simple "infidelity" in any meaningful sense than a scrupulous fealty to a deeply established if questionable family tradition, a pattern that seemed to include trying to go dad or grandad one or two better as time went on.

And while hardly happy about all this, the wives in the Kennedy family, as with Hillary Clinton, had their own secondary recompense. Like a spouse who stays and "suffers" with an alcoholic partner, there was tremendous public sympathy for the women much of the world saw as "cheated on." And, as also with Hillary, it was a sympathy few willingly gave up, Catholic prohibitions on divorce aside. Not till Ted and Joan split did the "D" word become active.

Then too, there is the enormous satisfaction of being able to say, as all the Kennedy wives could, "Yes, he's seeing *that woman* [as even Bill called Ms. Lewinsky]. But he's married to *me*." And such a statement is doubly satisfying when *that woman,* after all, is one of the most glamorous on the planet. It is a statement, incidentally, that several first ladies, including Eleanor Roosevelt and Mamie Eisenhower, have been able to make. It becomes rather hard to see such figures simply as "victims" and their husbands simply as "cads."

Thoughtful clinicians ought to similarly recognize that partners are occasionally set up for affairs. One case I recall involved a young couple married ten years, in which the wife–let's call her Jill–refused for all that time to have sex any more than once or twice a year. Despite pleading from the husband–we'll call him Bart–she likewise refused to attend therapy.

Meanwhile, friends of Jill and Bart–we'll call them Ernie and Pam– were heading for divorce. Ernie had become involved with another woman, and Pam had given him an ultimatum: she was going away to a wilderness cabin for a vacation. She'd return in a month, and he'd better have made up his mind to stay or leave.

Ernie, flushed with guilt, and also genuinely concerned about Pam's spending a month in a wilderness camp by herself, talked with Jill, and the two of them devised a plan: Bart, who loved the outdoors and whose fidelity to Jill despite her lack of physical intimacy with him "proved" he could be "trusted," would stay with Pam for the month in the cabin in the wilderness. Both Ernie and Jill thought their plan was splendid. Bart and Pam naively concurred.

Inevitably, in the month alone together in the wilderness, despite many attempts to restrain themselves, Bart and Pam, both love starved, became romantically and sexually involved. Ernie was delighted; Pam couldn't be mad at him any more, and he knew Bart would take care of her. Jill was also ultimately happy, though she was upset at first. But having wanted out of her marriage for many years, as she subsequently admitted to Bart, but afraid to be the one to leave, she'd gotten–unconsciously, one suspects–Bart and Pam to solve her problem for her. It was a perfect setup.

Such events aren't unusual. A good friend who had been involved in an extramarital relationship for several years, overburdened with guilt, one day confessed all to her husband. "I know," he said, in response to her *mea culpa*. "I've been trying to stay out of your way." Another friend described to me her parents' marriage, in which each had had retaliatory affairs for 20 years. If the wife slept with so and so, the husband got back at her by sleeping with one of her friends. The wife would sleep with someone else in revenge, and so on and so forth (drawing in a *heck* of a lot of other people, it would seem, and by definition, requiring basically *equal* numbers of men and women). Finally, they grew tired of the competition and stopped. Within months they got divorced. There was nothing holding them together anymore.

Again, let me try to be clear about my point. It certainly isn't that affairs are inherently good, or painless, or that researchers and therapists should encourage them. But affairs, like any relational behavior, invariably have important relational *functions* that scholars and clinicians ignore at our own and the public's peril, and we should stop treating them like robberies or sedition and try understanding them the same way we seek to understand other complex human phenomena. They are often, as the Kennedy experience shows, not largely about particular marriages, but about much older bonds. And as the other examples demonstrate, the "aggrieved party" may often be a conscious or unconscious instigator of them.

They don't necessarily tear couples apart, but can, ironically, as in the case of retaliatory involvements, be all that's holding them together. And, as almost any clinician who's worked for long with couples knows, they may help bring to the surface deeper problems that had lain neglected for years, and in so doing, may even have a positive effect on the primary dyadic union—a subject for another discussion.

And yet too often, we have the hardest time grasping such fairly obvious points. We must thus ask ourselves why.

WHY IT'S HARD TO THINK CLEARLY ABOUT AFFAIRS

So why do we think so foggily about these things? Why do people like us, who can run regression analyses and cite sources back decades from memory, find it so hard to grasp the most basic mathematical relationships when they're applied to "illicit" sex? Why do clinicians who seem otherwise to place great store in concepts such as "non-blaming" and "neutrality" often seem so eager, when it comes to affairs, to take sides?

Well, there are several possible answers. Here are a few of mine. We are still, at bottom, sexist about sex. We like to believe more men have affairs than women, and that individually men have affairs more frequently—which mathematically is impossible—because we still have trouble imagining women being attracted simply by sex, or imagining men having deep seated emotions. Yet surely we have heard enough about the Messalinas and the Wives of Bath, Catherine the Greats and Queen Charlottes and the "gay divorcees" and the "looking for Mr. Good Bars" of the world, surely we've heard Ray Charles sing "I Can't

Stop Loving You," enough to know that images of women as purely "emotional" and men as purely "physical" are obvious caricatures of who we are, not science.

And surely we should be able to see at some point that our own discomfort with our awareness of extradyadic unions, along with our halting attempts at explanations for them–like our tenuous suggestions that they happen "more" in modern life because women are "working more outside the home"–as if Strom Thurmond never fathered a child with his parents' maid in the 1920s or the postman never rang twice in the 1940s or people in Caligula's or Chaucer's time couldn't have had so many affairs because women "stayed at home"–that our patchwork explanations theories are often simply our own insecurity with a phenomenon we have barely begun to fathom causing us to grasp at straws.

Similarly, we separate physical sex and emotion from each other– something we would never do in any other context–or adopt clearly prejudiced labels for the people who are involved in them–out of our lack of understanding of affairs, perhaps even our fear that if we really simply analyzed them dispassionately some might accuse us of endorsing them, as further evidence of science's complicity in "the breakdown of marriage," as it often is called.

Frightened by this possibility, perhaps, we fail to remind ourselves that affairs have never "broken down" the institution of marriage, because if they had marriage would have ended eons ago. On the contrary, as commentators have for centuries reminded us, and as Spencer Tracy and Katherine Hepburn or simply our Aunt Matilda and her "friend" Mr. Smith should have taught us, some affairs, often enough, have made unbearable marriages bearable, supporting at least their form, if not always their heart.

My purpose in this paper is at bottom simply to urge us to take a step back from ourselves and our work, and try to look at things a little more disinterestedly than we might, to stop assuming that in examining extradyadic unions our goal is to do anything in particular about them, rather than try first of all to truly understand them; to survey less, perhaps, and to think about the surveys we have already done much more; to ask hard questions about our theories, our data, our terminology, and our goals.

The world has not collapsed because of extradyadic relationships, though plenty of people have been killed leaping to conclusions about them. Let us be sure we do not follow in their path, or help add to the toll.

REFERENCES

Gersen, R., & McGoldrick, M. (1985). *Genograms in family assessment*. New York: Norton.

Greeley, M., Micheal, R.T., & Smith, T.W. (1990). Americans and their sexual partners. *Society, 5,* 36-42.

Hansen, G.L. (1987). Extradyadic relations during courtship. *Journal of Sex Research, 23,* 382-390.

Lee, J. (1990). Lookin for love. In J. Lee's *Best of Johnny Lee* (compact disc). Warner Records: Nashville, TN.

Smith, T.W. (1991). Adult sexual behavior in 1989: Number of partners, frequency of intercourse, and risk of IADS. *Family Planning Perspectives, 23*(3), 102-107.

RESEARCH

Internet Infidelity:
A Multi-Phase Delphi Study

Tim Nelson
Fred P. Piercy
Douglas H. Sprenkle

Tim Nelson, PhD, is Coordinator, Marriage and Family Therapy Program, Bethel College, 1001 West McKinley Avenue, Mishawaka, IN 46545 (E-mail: nelsont@bethelcollege.edu).

Fred P. Piercy, PhD, is Professor of Family Therapy and Department Head, Department of Human Development, 366 Wallace, Virginia Polytechnic Institute and State University, Blacksburg, VA 24061-0416 (E-mail: piercy@vt.edu).

Douglas H. Sprenkle, PhD, is Professor of Family Therapy, Department of Child Development and Family Studies, 1269 Fowler House, Purdue University, West Lafayette, IN 47906 (E-mail: sprenkled@aol.com).

The authors would like to thank the following for their participation as expert panelists in this study: Michael Anderson; Robert Birch; Emily Brown; Rebecca Hope Dnistran; Marcus Earle; Shirley Glass; Erica Goodstone; Kristi Gordon; Terry Hargrave; Fred Humphrey; Julie Jurich; Ann Langley; Debbie Layton-Tholl; Don-David Lusterman; Frank Pittman; Cynthia Ruberg; Jennifer Schneider; Mark Schwartz; Terry Trepper; and Tom Wright.

[Haworth co-indexing entry note]: "Internet Infidelity: A Multi-Phase Delphi Study." Nelson, Tim, Fred P. Piercy, and Douglas H. Sprenkle. Co-published simultaneously in *Journal of Couple & Relationship Therapy* (The Haworth Press) Vol. 4, No. 2/3, 2005, pp. 173-194; and: *Handbook of the Clinical Treatment of Infidelity* (ed: Fred P. Piercy, Katherine M. Hertlein, and Joseph L. Wetchler) The Haworth Press, Inc., 2005, pp. 173-194. Single or multiple copies of this article are available for a fee from The Haworth Document Delivery Service [1-800-HAWORTH, 9:00 a.m. - 5:00 p.m. (EST). E-mail address: docdelivery@haworthpress.com].

Digital Object Identifier: 10.1300/J398v04n02_15

SUMMARY. We used a multi-phase Delphi methodology to identify and explore critical issues, interventions, and gender differences in the treatment of Internet infidelity. We developed three representative vignettes related to Internet infidelity and asked twenty experts in extramarital affairs and/or sex addiction to respond to them, both through ratings and open-ended comments. We found little agreement among the experts. We discuss the unique features of Internet relationships, the areas of agreement and disagreement that we found among the experts, and the implications of our findings and the nature of Internet infidelity for both practice and training in marriage and family therapy. *[Article copies available for a fee from The Haworth Document Delivery Service: 1-800-HAWORTH. E-mail address: <docdelivery@haworthpress.com> Website: <http://www.HaworthPress.com> © 2005 by The Haworth Press, Inc. All rights reserved.]*

KEYWORDS. Internet infidelity, extramarital affairs, Delphi methodology, treatment strategies, relational issues

Within the last decade, the rise in popularity of the Internet has led to an ever-increasing number of spouses meeting others, outside of their marriage, in chat rooms. Many of these relationships start off innocently and end after a short period of time. However, an alarming number develop into emotional and/or physical extramarital affairs (Glass, 2000, personal communication). This phenomenon is referred to as Internet infidelity.

By now most MFTs have seen cases of Internet infidelity in their practice. We define Internet infidelity as using the Internet to take sexual energy of any sort–thoughts, feelings, and behaviors–outside of a committed sexual relationship in such a way that it damages the relationship. It is further exacerbated when one spouse pretends that this drain of energy will affect neither their partner nor the relationship, as long as it remains undiscovered. Although lustful thoughts and feelings outside of a marriage are not inherently harmful or wrong, acting on these feelings and/or hiding them devitalizes the relationship, compromises integrity, and co-opts the other partner's choices (Shaw, 1997).

Historically, husbands have been more likely to have extramarital affairs. However, increasing numbers of women also begin and participate in extramarital affairs (Laumann et al., 1994). This trend could be said to be the result of the women's movement, increased participation of women in the workforce, and/or more liberal sexual attitudes for women in our culture. However, the emergence of the Internet has made it increasingly easy for both spouses to become involved in extramarital affairs. Estimates by Nua (2000) indicate that there are currently over 275.54 million people using the Internet worldwide, with 136.06 million of these users in the U.S. and Canada. If the estimate is that only one percent of all of these people are looking for love on their computers, that means nearly 13 million adults could be directly impacted.

To date, we know little about how therapists are handling cases of Internet infidelity. Clearly, the context under which Internet affairs occur is different than the "traditional" extramarital affair. The Internet has several characteristics which make it the ideal medium for sexual involvement. It is widely accessible, inexpensive, legal, available in the privacy of one's own home, anonymous, and also generally does not put the user at direct risk of contracting a sexually-transmitted disease (Cooper, 1999). Marriage and family therapists need guidance in how to assess and address the unique challenges of Internet infidelity.

Hence, the purpose of this study was to determine how experts in the fields of sex addiction and/or extramarital affairs treat cases of Internet infidelity in their practice. We hoped that, in identifying areas of expert agreement, we could determine more effective methods of handling this unique issue in therapy.

Assumptions

This study is based on the following assumptions:

1. Internet infidelity requires specific clinical expertise if it is to be handled appropriately by marriage and family therapists;
2. There are specific critical issues, interventions, and gender differences within cases of Internet infidelity that, when clarified, will enhance the clinical work of MFTs who work with these special cases;
3. The feminist critique of family therapy has influenced the field to the degree that any gender differences in cases of Internet infidelity will be approached judiciously; and
4. The Delphi methodology, which tabulates the collective thinking of a knowledgeable panel of experts in a field, is a relevant methodology to perform exploratory investigations on how to best serve couples and families struggling with the issue of Internet infidelity.

The Marriage of the Internet and Infidelity

Hammersley (1995), has speculated on a number of reasons why people find Internet sex and communication so appealing. These include the fact that: people can easily communicate with others whom they would normally never meet; communication costs are low; people can download software toys and games which are reinforcing; people can keep in touch with minimal time; people are taken seriously and listened to; and people can present a different persona, which may deviate in significant ways from one's everyday, face-to-face persona if they so choose. Indeed, sex in "cyberspace" offers yet another vehicle through which individuals in unhappy marriages can express (and act on) their emotional loneliness or sexual fantasies.

Furthermore, computer relationships also can offer a certain degree of anonymity and safety (Lebow, 1998). This anonymity allows intense intimacy to develop between people in a very short time. Many participants in computer relationships that began on-line feel that their relationship is truly unique–that it grew from the inside-out, instead of outside– in as face-to-face relationships do (Schnarch, 1997). Leiblum (1997) explains that the Internet is a virtual, painless, risk-free, other-centered substitute for the pain, responsibility, and reality of a true relationship. For couples whose marriage is already vulnerable, this outlet can provide the ingredients and context for the beginnings of an extramarital affair.

Moreover, consistent with Hammersley (1995), there is no opportunity on-line for one to compare a partner's self-presentation to what one might experience in person. There is no opportunity for a person to look deeply into the other–which is partly what makes Internet relationships so alluring (Schnarch, 1997). Sex on the Internet is like having an affair because people often do things with less important partners–or when they are anonymous–that they cannot do with their own spouse. That is, some disgruntled spouses seek outlets for their eroticism and loneliness on the Internet in ways they cannot within their primary relationship. They seek gratification through the Internet because they believe it will not jeopardize acceptance from their primary partner.

Finally, sex and power in relationships have been traditionally repressive for women who have had to acquiesce to male dominance because, in most instances, they have not been on a level playing field in those societies (Carter, 1996). Women have not found many outlets for their sexuality; neither have they been allowed to explore channels to power through their sexuality (Roadway, 1989). In recent studies of romance readers, Roadway (1992) found that women enjoy romance erotica because it provides a vicarious sense of power and satisfaction. Yet, this type of expression is not reciprocal. Internet sex, on the other hand, offers women a chance to both give and receive pleasure. This forum allows the woman to have an interactive experience both in the creation of the text and through control of the story. The reader, creator, and text are linked in an unending erotic exchange that is highly alluring for women caught in a stale, lifeless marriage (Roadway, 1992).

Consequences of Internet Infidelity

Schneider (2000), conducted a survey of 91 women and 3 men, aged 24-57, who had experienced serious adverse consequences because of their partner's cybersex involvements. In 60.6% of cases, the sexual activities were limited to cybersex and did not include off-line sex. And although not specifically asked about this, 31% of her subjects revealed that the cybersex activities were a continuation of pre-existing compulsive sexual behaviors. Open-ended questions also yielded the following conclusions: (a) In response to learning about their partner's on-line sexual activities, the survey respondents felt hurt, betrayal, rejection, abandonment, devastation, loneliness, shame, isolation, humiliation, jealousy, and anger, as well as loss of self-esteem. Being lied to repeatedly was a major cause of distress; (b) Cybersex addiction was a major contributing factor to the eventual separation and divorce of the couples within this survey: 22.3% of the respondents were separated or divorced, and several others were seriously contemplating leaving; (c) Among 68% of the couples, one or both had lost interest in relational sex: 52.1% of addicts had decreased interest in sex with their spouse, as did 34% of partners. Some couples had had no relational sex in months or years; (d) Partners compared themselves unfavorably with the on-line women (or men) and pictures, and felt hopeless about being able to compete with them; (e) Partners overwhelmingly felt that cyber affairs were as emotionally painful to them as "live" or "off-line" affairs, and many believed that virtual affairs were just as much adultery or "cheating" as live affairs; and (f) Adverse effects on the children included: (1) exposure to "cyberporn" and to the objectification of women; (2) involvement in parental conflicts; (3) lack of attention because of one parent's involvement with the computer and the other parent's preoccupation with the cybersex addict; and (4) the negative effects of the eventual breakup of the marriage.

Treatment Strategies for Internet Infidelity

Currently, we know little about how MFTs or other mental health professionals treat cases of Internet infidelity in their practices. However, the extant research does provide some general direction and guidelines on how to treat these special cases in therapy.

For example, Schnarch (1997), as stated previously, holds that electronic relationships promote emotionally disconnected or superficially erotic contacts. He takes issue with the approach of using the Internet as a relationship skill development tool. He believes that clients are not practicing the self-confrontation, self-validation, and self-soothing skills they need. Instead they are avoiding confronting and maintaining who they want to be in their relationships.

Moreover, Schnarch (1997), contends that for the last decade pop psychologies have pandered to clients' anxieties, enshrined their fears, (e.g., of abandonment) and emphasized safety and security and acceptance as overriding principles. In this light, the Internet's virtues of anonymous contact without rejection or vulnerability and information without anxiety are provocatively inviting. And the Internet offers the same promise many therapies do–that, given the right information/technology, there are ways around your problems so you don't have to go through them. Using the Internet as a "baby step" approach to developing relationship skills also puts the focus on anxiety reduction rather than anxiety tolerance (differentiation), which is vital to keeping sex and intimacy alive in long-term relationships, according to Schnarch. In other words, an Internet relationship may approximate a real relationship–but, then, "so does sex with an inflatable doll." Neither one is likely to help people develop substantial capacity for an intimate relationship when they are subtly capitalizing on ways the one differs from the real thing (Schnarch, 1997, p. 19).

Analogously, Shaw (1997) maintains that it is crucial that the therapist respect the potential for stagnancy (and growth) already imposed by secrecy, disengagement, fusion, lack of differentiation, and underdeveloped integrity. She believes that therapists can avoid stagnancy by not holding the secrets of one partner from the other. She advocates that therapists meet conjointly with couples, rather than with either partner alone. This serves to help the relationship contain (instead of disperse) emotional energy, use it for growth, and put healthy boundaries around the marriage.

Treatment Strategies for Relational Issues and the Internet

Turkle (1995) believes that clinicians who recognize the complexity of on-line interactions can help their clients make positive use of electronic relating. Turkle contends that clients can use therapy to help them integrate the confidence and social dexterity they experience on-line into their everyday lives; to integrate rather than split off, those various aspects of themselves. As one individual in his study put it,

> I feel very different on-line. I am a lot more outgoing, less inhibited. I would say I feel more like myself. But that's a contradiction. I feel more like who I wish I was. I'm just hoping that face-to-face in my personal relationships, I can find a way to spend some time being the on-line me. (Turkle, 1995, p. 179)

Similarly, Cooper and Sportolari (1997) hold that Internet relationships reduce the role that physical attributes play in the development of attraction and instead enhance other factors such as proximity, rapport, similarity, and mutual self-disclosure, thus promoting erotic connections that stem from emotional intimacy rather than lustful attraction. They believe that the Internet is a model of intimate, yet separate relating. It allows adult (and teen) men and women more freedom to deviate from typically constraining gender roles that are often automatically activated in face-to-face relationships.

To this end, Cooper and Sportolari (1997), recommend that therapists tell their clients to go on-line as an adjunct to treatment. They hypothesize that clients who might benefit from going on-line in conjunction with their therapeutic exploration include, spouses and clients who are shy or avoidant, who are recovering from sexual assaults, who have difficulty integrating sexuality and intimacy, or who want to explore their sexual orientation or gender identity.

Lebow (1997) also urges therapists not to steer their clients from Internet communication, but that: (a) chat groups and news groups are not a substitute for therapy; (b) therapists should understand this territory and provide guidance to those who use these resources; (c) access to psychoeducation sites for information for families must also be provided; and (d) therapists must judiciously choose discussion groups as they can be used for support, information and connection with others who share a common interest or problem (e.g., infertility, raising children, or quadriplegia) but all are not equally as helpful.

Finally, Maheu and Subotnik (2001), in their book *Infidelity and the Internet* recommend that therapists first help clients cope and make sense of the emotions that attend Internet infidelity. They then work to help partners understand one another and develop more effective communication skills. And in their final stage, they work to reconstruct the broken trust and create a shared vision with the couple of what their new relationship should look like.

METHOD

Selection of the panelists for this Delphi study was of crucial importance to the success of the study. In choosing panelists, we considered certain criteria. Potential panelists needed to have at least two of the following five criteria:

1. published at least two refereed journal articles or one book on the topic of extramarital affairs or sex addiction;
2. had five or more years of clinical experience and seen at least five cases involving extramarital affairs or sex addiction
3. had five or more years of teaching experience in the field of extramarital affairs or sex addiction;
4. supervised or meta-vised at least five cases involving extramarital affairs or sex addiction; and
5. conducted at least one or more state, regional, or national convention presentations on extramarital affairs or sex addiction.

We generated expert panelists by investigating therapy and sex related refereed journals and books and selected authors who wrote about extramarital affairs or sex addiction and the Internet. Those panelists who chose to participate from the first list were also asked to generate names of other therapists or researchers who met the criteria listed above. We identified and selected a total of 20 (10 men and 10 women) experts in the field of extramarital affairs and sex addiction.

Procedures

Phase one of this study involved contacting, via e-mail and U.S. mail, 78 clinical members of the American Association of Marriage and Family Therapy. This list of members was obtained and purchased through the AAMFT list-serve. These 78 members were randomly selected from a larger list of 1,000 clinical members across the country. These members were asked to share the following information:

1. (a) Have you seen couples in your therapy where one or both partners is using the Internet for sexual satisfaction that is troubling to their partner? (b) Please describe the situation.
2. What, specifically, was troublesome for the "offended" partner?
3. How was it resolved (e.g., divorce, reconciliation, still in therapy, etc.)? A total of 36% of the respondents shared cases that they had seen or were currently seeing in their therapy.

Phase two involved examining each of the respondents' replies to determine the themes involving Internet infidelity among the clients of these clinical members of the AAMFT. Each case description was analyzed inductively (Patton, 1990) to derive themes across cases.

Phase three involved the creation of three representative vignettes from the themes that emerged from the responses of the clinical members. These vignettes are below.

Vignette A

A professional couple reports to you for marital therapy. The wife works from a computer out of their home where she became involved in a relationship with another person of the opposite sex. The husband knew nothing about the relationship. The husband found out about it through an old e-mail that was left in their garbage. The e-mail was flirtatious in nature and very uncharacteristic of how the wife behaves in their marriage. The husband is furious that his wife is communicating at this level of intimacy with a stranger. The third party also lives in a neighboring state and the husband does not believe that they have not been seeing each other. The wife explains that this was an outlet for her and is not the cause of their marital difficulties.

Vignette B

A married couple of eight years, with three children, comes to you for marital therapy. The husband is a frequent user of the Internet. He admits to you that he met another woman in a chat room and they began a relationship over the phone and through e-mail. Reluctantly, the husband also admits that he met with the third party on two separate occasions where they had sexual intercourse. The husband is scared, confused, and does not know if he wants to return to his marriage. The wife is extremely angry at the betrayal and is worried about the future of her family.

Vignette C

A couple comes to you for therapy after the husband is "caught" downloading pornographic material from various websites. The wife is outraged and disgusted by his "perversity and betrayal." She cannot understand why he "needs" to use pornography. The husband is embarrassed and ashamed about getting caught. The wife now does not trust his faithfulness to their marriage. The husband feels "It's no big deal. All guys do it."

Phase four involved distributing these vignettes to the 20 experts in the field of extramarital affairs and/or sex addiction. Panelists were asked to read each of the vignettes and to respond, in writing or over the phone, to the following questions:

1. Based upon the information given in this vignette, what do you believe are the critical issues that need to be addressed by therapists working with this couple/family?
2. What interventions would you use to address these critical issues in your therapy?
3. If the genders of the participants were changed within the vignette, how might your approach in therapy change?

Eight of the experts were interviewed over the phone. This procedure allowed the researcher to gather data and clarify any ambiguous statements directly with the expert panelist. Each of the remaining twenty panelists responded by electronic mail.

Phase five involved calling four of the expert panelists who provided unconventional or ambiguous statements through electronic mail. These conversations provided the researcher with the rationale and clarifications necessary for the other panelists to evaluate and respond to one another's answers.

In phase six, the responses from each of the experts were then analyzed inductively to derive themes across responses. Each non-overlapping response for all panelists was included in the phase six questionnaire. Rather than eliminating redundant responses from each of the panelists, all related issues were included under the broader "critical issues," "interventions" and "gender differences" for each category.

We edited responses for clarity and redundancy and made every effort to retain the wording and meaning of the original items. We grouped the responses into three categories: "critical issues," "interventions" and "gender differences." The rationale for confusing and/or ambiguous responses was also recorded for review and response by the other experts. One doctoral student and two faculty members read through the responses to ensure accuracy, clarity, and non-redundancy.

In the seventh and final phase, participants were asked to log on to a website, and then to read, rate, and respond to each of the responses on a Likert scale (1 = Strongly Disagree to 7 = Strongly Agree). Participants were also instructed to read the rationale for any confusing/ambiguous responses to which they had concerns. A similar option was also provided for any related issues subsumed under the broader "critical issue," "intervention," or "gender difference." These rationales and related issues were "hyperlinked" to the specific items with which they were associated. Participants were given the option to directly respond on the website to each of the rationale and/or responses of the other experts. This provided a qualitative iteration to the Delphi.

Items on the final questionnaires were analyzed to calculate medians and interquartile ranges. Medians and interquartile ranges identify the rates of group agreement and consensus for each item. The medians and interquartile ranges were used to compile responses to questions into three response profiles. These three response profiles are Profile 1: (a) items that met the criteria and were included in the final profile (median = 6.0 or greater; IQR = less than 1.50; Tables 2 and 3); Profile 2: (b) items that did not meet the criteria for the final profile, but which were in close range (median = 5.50-5.9; IQR = 1.51-1.75; Tables 4, 5, and 6).

Results of Final Phase of Delphi Study (Phase Six)

A total of 70% of the expert panelists responded to all three of the vignette questionnaires in phase six; while 80% answered the questionnaire for Vignette A only. The following series of tables (Tables 1-3) represent items that met the criteria for the 3 profiles of the study.

DISCUSSION

First Assumption

Surprisingly, the first assumption that Internet infidelity requires specific clinical expertise if it is to be handled appropriately by marriage

TABLE 1. Items from *Vignette A* That Met the Criteria for Inclusion in Final Profile 1A

(Median = 6.0 or greater; IQR 1.50 or less)

ITEM	MEDIAN	IQR
Critical Issues		
#6. The violation of marital trust and the betrayal................................	7.0	0.00

TABLE 2. Items from *Vignette B* That Met the Criteria for Inclusion in Final Profile 1B

(Median = 6.0 or greater; IQR 1.50 or less)

ITEM	MEDIAN	IQR
Critical Issues		
#2. The wife's feelings of pain, fear, and betrayal..............................	7.00	0.00
Interventions		
#12. Use the affair to create a better union if this is what they choose...	7.00	1.00

TABLE 3. Items from *Vignette C* That Met the Criteria for Inclusion in Final Profile 1C

(Median = 6.0 or greater; IQR 1.50 or less)

ITEM	MEDIAN	IQR
Critical Issues		
#2. The therapist must not go into a state of moral outrage.................	7.00	1.50

TABLE 4. Items from *Vignette A* That Did Not Meet the Criteria for Inclusion in Final Profile 1, but Were in Close Range: Profile 2A

(Median = 5.50 -5.59; IQR = 1.51-1.75.)

ITEM	MEDIAN	IQR
Interventions	6.50	1.75
#1. Do a complete relationship history...		
#2. Work to create an atmosphere where they can feel safe enough with each other to tell the truth...	7.0	1.75

and family therapists, was not supported by the data. It appears as if the ease of starting and continuing an extramarital relationship through the Internet is not necessarily important when treating cases of Internet infidelity, according to this group of expert panelists. This was the result even though each of the vignettes represented different degrees of involvement by the involved spouse.

TABLE 5. Items from *Vignette B* That Did Not Meet the Criteria for Inclusion in Final Profile 1, but Were in Close Range: Profile 2B

(Median = 5.50-5.59; IQR = 1.51-1.75)

ITEM	MEDIAN	IQR
Critical Issues		
#14. Development of trust again...	7.00	1.75

TABLE 6. Items from *Vignette C* That Did Not Meet the Criteria for Inclusion in Final Profile 1, but Were in Close Range: Profile 2C

(Median = 5.50-5.59; IQR = 1.51-1.75)

ITEM	MEDIAN	IQR
Critical Issues		
#19. Is the husband understanding his own problem and dealing with his embarrassment and shame..	6.00	1.75

Apparently, the context through which the infidelity develops, as well as the level of involvement, are seen as more "symptomatic" issues of the underlying problem. In support of this, one panelist stated, "The fact that the relationship began on the Internet makes no difference to me. I treat these kinds of cases in therapy the same as if they met the third party in a bar or at work." Similarly, another told us, "I don't deal with these Internet cases any differently. The fact that it began on the Internet is not the issue for me." Still another expert said, "The computer and the Internet is not the issue."

Why the experts did not see the Internet as an important variable within each of the vignettes is unclear. We could surmise that they do not view these relationships differently from "traditional" cases of infidelity because research has not been conducted that confirms that they are, in fact, different. As stated previously, little is known about Internet infidelity since, to date, there has only been one study done on this topic (Schneider, 2000).

Furthermore, existing literature supports the fact that across "traditional" cases of extramarital infidelity contextual variables such as place, time, and circumstance are generally not seen as critical issues in the assessment and treatment of infidelity. For example, Pittman (1989) believes that the identity of the third party and how they met are not the key issues to address in therapy. Rather, he maintains that therapy must focus upon the individual and his or her specific faulty decision making processes that left him or her vulnerable to external temptations. Pittman maintains that you cannot remove all of the possible temptations from an individual's environment. Hence, focusing on these issues in therapy is a futile endeavor.

Second Assumption

The second assumption of this study was also not well supported by the results. This assumption was that there are specific critical issues, interventions, and gender differences within cases of Internet infidelity that, when clarified, will enhance the clinical work of MFTs who work with these special cases. In fact, there were only a total of four items (out of the 176 from all three vignettes) that had both strong agreement and consensus. And only four of the other items were in close range. The medians and interquartile ranges on the remainder of items either lacked sufficient agreement and consensus to be included in the final profiles or the results were largely disparate, indicating panelist divisiveness. Hence, from the data of this study, it is not clear whether there are, in fact, specific critical issues, interventions, and gender differences in cases of Internet infidelity that need to be addressed in therapy.

It is difficult to know why there was not greater consensus and agreement on a larger percentage of the items. It could be that the divisiveness that existed in this study reflects the divisiveness that currently exists in the extant literature. Indeed, a tenable argument could be made that the divisiveness that already exists in how to best treat "traditional" cases of extramarital infidelity is analogous to the divisiveness that was found in how to treat cases of Internet infidelity. The Internet only seems to add another, more convenient, mechanism through which an extramarital affair can begin and be sustained.

In fact, a large percentage of the truly divisive items in this study could be categorized under five specific areas that are already debated in the existing literature. These five topics include:

1. How should therapists handle secrets in cases of extramarital infidelity?
2. Should the therapist take a more individual or relational approach in cases of extramarital infidelity?
3. What amount and type of disclosure is helpful for the noninvolved spouse to know?
4. Should the noninvolved spouse monitor the involved spouse's behavior?
5. Which specific theoretical and treatment approaches are most helpful in the treatment of extramarital infidelity?

Third Assumption: Possible Interpretations

There appeared to be marginal support for the third assumption of this study as well. This assumption was that the feminist critique of family therapy has influenced the field to the degree that any gender differences in cases of Internet infidelity will be approached judiciously. A variety of explanations could be offered to explain the divisiveness on these items. Two are offered below.

First, it could be that many of the differences in paradigm that existed within this panel could be attributed to their epistemology. The development of any philosophical paradigm comes from one's epistemological source: authority, intuition, reasoning, and/or experience (Jones & Butman, 1991). Some of the comments made by many of the panelists were based upon their own personal or clinical experiences, while others emphasized the findings of research. These differences in epistemological source might account for the divisiveness on these items as the clinical and personal experiences of one expert may have differed from the research findings and interpretations of others.

Furthermore, the challenges of the feminist critique of family therapy also may not have been a part of the training or knowledge base of many of these experts. A number of the panelists within this study were likely trained during an era when modernism was the prevailing clinical zeitgeist. However, due to the fact that the data within this study were not analyzed according to the age, gender, or theoretical orientation of the panelist, it is difficult to know whether this is a tenable hypothesis or not. Further research that asks experts to identify whether or not they claim a feminist clinical orientation would help to clarify these suppositions.

Hence, it could be surmised that the epistemology as well as the training of the panelists influenced their responses to these items. However, it is crucial to emphasize that these hypotheses are only tentative and that other, perhaps more tenable, assertions could also be made to explain the divisiveness that existed in this study.

DISCUSSION, ANALYSIS, AND REFLECTIONS

The findings of this study were indeed intriguing and perhaps even counter-intuitive in many respects. First, none of the experts saw the Internet as being an important contextual variable in any of the vignettes. Second, it was curious that the experts were unable to agree on all but a few items across the three vignettes. Finally, it was intriguing that there was such divisiveness across so many of the items. A brief analysis and reflection on each of these issues follows.

The findings of this study indicate that the panelists did not see the Internet as an important contextual variable in cases of Internet infidelity. Not one expert even mentioned the Internet as a critical issue within any of the vignettes. This finding is counter to the clinical research of Cooper (2002), Schnarch (1997), and Shaw (1997), who maintain that these cases do require special clinical knowledge. For example, Cooper (2002), theorizes that Internet infidelity is indeed a unique type of extramarital affair due to the anonymity, accessibility, and affordability or the Internet. Furthermore, as mentioned earlier, Schnarch (1997) argues that the Internet lends itself to maximum self-presentation by commission and omission. Indeed, Schnarch believes that the Internet is a relatively poor stimulus for the self-confrontation and the core disclosure that epitomize intense intimacy–which, in part, explains its popularity as a social network.

It is also important to note that simply because many of the specific critical issues, interventions and gender differences did not have strong consensus and agreement within this study, does not necessarily mean that they still are not important in therapy. Indeed, a number of the experts indicated in their comments that even though some of the other issues and interventions listed were important, they would not choose to privilege them in their therapy. The data in this study also support these assertions in that a substantial number of the items that did not make either of the first two profiles still had strong agreement scores. Indeed, a larger number of items could have been included in the strong agreement and consensus profiles had the criteria for inclusion been less stringent.

Finally, it is also critical to emphasize that the vast majority of the extant literature on extramarital affairs is clinical research. We still have little empirical data that verifies such concepts as affair typologies, much less which kinds of interventions are most effective in treating cases of extramarital infidelity in therapy. Hence, the divisiveness that existed in this study could largely be due to the fact that many prominent theorists and clinicians will disagree about a variety of clinical issues due to the lack of definitive research on these issues.

Future research in this area should provide more clues as to whether or not Internet infidelity is, in fact, different from "traditional" cases of extramarital infidelity. This research will also hopefully help us find more clues about what are the specific critical issues, interventions and gender differences that therapists must address to effectively treat cases of Internet infidelity. This research will be especially important during this challenging time of managed care, when limited therapy session allotments are often the norm and therapists are asked to provide treatments that are proven to be effective.

Implications for the MFT Field, MFT Training, and Clinical Practice

There are a variety of implications for the field of MFT both from the qualitative results of this study, and from the unique features of Internet relationships. The following eight implications are recommended for MFT training and clinical practice.

1. Clearly this study emphasized the enormous amount of knowledge that is helpful for therapists to know when treating cases of Internet infidelity (i.e., there were a total 176 distinctly different critical issues, interventions and gender differences mentioned by panelists across the 3 vignettes). Moreover, the study illustrated that there is still no one "right way" of conducting therapy for those engaged in Internet infidelity. The divisiveness within this study emphasized the fact that the large number of different theoretical orientations across the field leaves therapists with a variety of treatment options for cases of infidelity. MFT trainers would be well served to continue stressing self-of-the-therapist issues (Aponte, 1991) with beginning therapists so that issues of epistemology, paradigm and theory are clear. Indeed, the "right" answers will be determined through future research and/or through

further discussions related to the important issue of Internet infidelity.

2. MFT training and curricula in religious values, morals, ethical issues and how to address them in therapy should also become a target of training in graduate MFT programs. Cases of infidelity highlight the link between morality and therapy. Therapists may have certain basic beliefs about marital infidelity that will guide their thinking in working with those who have experienced an extramarital infidelity. It is important that therapists are clear about their views on these issues. Inevitably, therapists will have to address questions concerning their own values and beliefs about affairs: Are affairs always wrong? If there has been an affair does that mean there must be a separation or divorce? Can someone be in love with more than one person at one time? It is vital that therapists are clear on where they stand on these issues so that clients can be duly informed.

3. MFTs must continue to emphasize the maintenance stage of change (Prochaska & DiClemente, 1982, 1983) with cases of Internet infidelity. That is, it will be important to help clients maintain faithfulness, if that is their goal, since the temptation to start another affair will be greater because of one's accessibility to a partner through the Internet.

4. Studies point to attraction being highest when the partner is perceived as being both physically attractive and attitudinally similar to oneself (Brehm, 1992). The Internet increases one's chances of connecting with like-minded people due to the computer's ability to rapidly sort along many dimensions simultaneously. Indeed, an attitude is being promulgated that says, "Life will be happier for the online individual because the people with whom one interacts most strongly will be selected more by commonality of interests and goals than by accidents of proximity" (Lichlider cited in Rheingold, 1993, p. 24). The implications of these findings are that Internet infidelity cases could be more insidious to marriages as Internet partners may have an appeal that is greater than the "traditional" affair partner. MFTs will need to be particularly vigilant of the power and attraction that Internet relationships have upon spouses who have strayed.

5. One of the significant findings within this study was that experts agreed that affairs can be used to create a stronger marriage, if this is what both partners choose. In support of this,

Glass and Wright (1992, 1997) offer several questions that therapists might raise to help couples recover from an infidelity. These include questions such as: (a) What decision making processes did the involved spouse employ as s/he was deciding to engage in the infidelity? (b) What are both spouses' attitudes and beliefs about infidelity now? (c) What needs were being met by the extramarital relationship that may be compensating for perceived inadequacies in the marriage? (d) What role did the involved spouse take in the extramarital relationship that makes him or her feel bad as well as good about himself or herself? and (e) What growth or insights, developed through this extramarital relationship, can be shared or integrated back into the marriage relationship?

6. The findings of this study confirm the fact that paying attention to the emotions of the clients who are struggling with an infidelity is essential. Thus, training in relationship skills is crucial for novice therapists in that these skills are the foundation upon which all other techniques and skills are built (Asay & Lambert, 1999). New therapists need to be taught how to be effective and supportive listeners; how to create meaningful dialogue with clients; how to build effective therapeutic alliances; how to monitor therapeutic alliances; and how to repair torn alliances. Therapists particularly need special training and skills so as not to form unhealthy coalitions with either spouse in cases of extramarital infidelity.

7. The results of this study indicate that couples can and do recover from extramarital affairs. It is the responsibility of MFTs to continue to encourage and foster a sense of hope to individuals who want to restore their marriage but are beleaguered by the work that is necessary to achieve this.

8. The results of this study also confirm the fact that the arrival of the Internet challenges therapists to become even more proficient in helping couples to develop boundaries around their marriage. With the development of the Internet, therapists will be needed to help couples draw these boundaries in this uncharted area (Shapiro, 1997). Glass (1997, 2000, personal communication) also suggests some helpful ways of keeping Internet infidelity in check: include your spouse in any chat rooms you enter while on the Internet just as you would if you went to a party together; let your spouse know about the development of any friendships on the Internet; and spend more time

together with your spouse than you do with relative strangers on the Internet.

CONCLUSION

The Internet is pervasive and here to stay. MFTs will be well served to recognize the Internet as a powerful medium with the potential to re-shape relationships and to restructure our social world (Cooper & Sportolari, 1997). Clearly, the Internet offers many positives. It provides a medium for immediate and discreet delivery of information and companionship to those in need. However, it is by no means a mature medium. The Internet can be a minefield for a naïve user and perhaps an irresistible temptation to a lonely spouse. Therapists, especially ones who deal with marriage, will be needed as more and more couples find themselves dealing with an Internet infidelity.

This study underscores the divisiveness even among experts about the difficulties inherent in treating cases of Internet infidelity in therapy. We also hope that MFTs will begin to clarify how the Internet can be used as a medium of healthy connection and restoration for the couples we serve.

REFERENCES

Aponte, H. (1994). *Bread and spirit: Therapy with the new poor.* New York: Norton.

Carter, B. (1996). *Love, honor, and negotiate: Making your marriage work.* New York: Simon and Schuster.

Glass, S.P., & Wright, T.L. (1977). The relationship of extramarital sex, length of marriage, and sex differences on marital satisfaction and romanticism: Athanasiou's data reanalyzed. *Journal of Marriage and the Family, 39,* 691-703.

Glass, S.P., & Wright, T.L. (1987). Sex differences in type of extramarital involvement and marital dissatisfaction. *Sex Roles, 12,* 1101-1119.

Glass, S.P., & Wright, T.L. (1985). Clinical implications of research on extramarital involvement. In R.A. Brown, and J.R. Field (Eds.), *Treatment of sexual problems in individuals and couples therapy.* New York: PMA Publishing Corporation.

Glass, S.P., & Wright, T.L. (1988). Clinical implications of research on extramarital involvement. In R. Brown & J. Field (Eds.), *Treatment of sexual problems in individual and couples therapy.* New York: PMA.

Glass, S.P., & Wright, T.L. (1992). Justifications for extramarital relationships: The association between attitudes, behaviors, and gender. *The Journal of Sex Research, 29,* 361- 387.

Glass, S.P., & Wright, T.L. (1997). Reconstructing marriages after the trauma of infidelity. In K. Halford & H.J. Markman (Eds.), *Clinical handbook of marriage and couples interventions* (pp. 471-507). New York: John Wiley & Sons.

Jones, S.L., & Butman, R.E. (1991). *Modern psychotherapies: A comprehensive Christian appraisal*. Illinois: Intervarsity Press.

Laumann, E.O., Gagnon, J.H. Michael, R.T., & Michaels, S. (1994). *The social organization of sexuality: Sexual practices in the United States*. Chicago: University of Chicago Press.

Lebow, J. (1998). Not just talk, maybe some risk: The therapeutic potentials and pitfalls of computer-mediated conversation. *Journal of Marital and Family Therapy, 24*, 203-206.

Leiblum, S.R. (1997). Sex and the net: Clinical implications. *Journal of Sex Education & Therapy, 22*, 21-28.

Lusterman, D.D. (1998). *Infidelity: A survival guide*. Oakland, CA: New Harbinger Publications.

Lusterman, D. (1995). Treating marital infidelity. In R. H. Mikesell, D. Lusterman, & S.H. McDaniel (Eds.), *Integrating family therapy: Handbook of family psychology and systems theory*. Washington, DC: American Psychological Association.

Patton, M.Q. (1990). *Qualitative evaluation and research methods: 2nd edition*. California: Sage.

Pittman, F.S. (1987). *Turning points: Treating families in crisis*. New York: W.W. Norton.

Pittman, F.S. (1989). *Private lies: Infidelity and the betrayal of intimacy*. New York: W.W. Norton.

Pittman, F. (1991). The secret passions of men. *The Journal of Marital and Family Therapy, 17*, 11-23.

Pittman, F.S., & Wagers, T.P. (1992). *Crisis of infidelity*. In A.S. Gurman and N. Jacobsen (Eds.), *In clinical handbook of couple therapy*. New York: Guilford.

Prochaska, J.O., & DiClemente, C.C. (1983). Stages and processes of self-change of smoking: Toward an integrative model of change. *Journal of Consulting and Clinical Psychology, 51*, 390-395.

Roadway, J. (1984). *Reading the romance: Women, patriarchy, and popular literature*. Chapel Hill, NC: University of North Carolina Press.

Schnarch, D. (1991). *Constructing the sexual crucible*. New York: W.W. Norton & Company.

Schnarch, D. (1997). *Passionate marriage*. New York: W.W. Norton & Company.

Schnarch, D. (1997). Sex, intimacy, and the Internet. *Journal of Sex Education and Therapy, 22*, 15-20.

Schneider, J.P. (1988). *Back from betrayal: Recovering from his affairs*. Center City, MN: Hazelden Educational Materials.

Schneider, J.P., & Schneider, B. (1990). *Sex, lies, and forgiveness: Couples speak on healing from sex addiction*. Center City, MN: Hazelden Educational Materials.

Schneider, J.P. (1994). Sex addiction: Controversy within mainstream addiction medicine, diagnosis based on the DSM-III-R, and physician case histories. *Sexual Addiction & Compulsivity, 1*, 19-44.

Schneider, J.P. (2000). Effects of cybersex addiction on the family: Results of a survey. *Sexual Addiction and Compulsivity, 2*, 12-33.

194 HANDBOOK OF THE CLINICAL TREATMENT OF INFIDELITY

Shapiro, A. (1997). Fantasy affairs or dangerous liaisons? Relationships in the cyber-world. *Family Therapy News, 2*, 12-14.

Shaw, J. (1997). Treatment rationale for Internet infidelity. *Journal of Sex Education and Therapy, 22*, 29-34.

Subotnik, R., & Harris, G. (1994). *Surviving infidelity*. Holbrook, MA: Bob Adams Press.

Turkle, S. (1995). *Life on the screen*. New York: Simon and Schuster.

Assessing the Relationship
Between Differentiation and Infidelity:
A Structural Equation Model

Katherine M. Hertlein
Gary Skaggs

SUMMARY. Differentiation and infidelity have been theoretically related. However, few studies have tested whether the concepts in differentiation are statistically related to infidelity. One hundred nineteen participants
in the present study completed two inventories assessing their level of differentiation and engaging in infidelity. Two-step structural equation modeling is used to determine the degree to which differentiation relates to
infidelity. Results indicated that, though differentiation may be part of a

---

Katherine M. Hertlein, MS, is Adjunct Faculty, Virginia Tech, 840 University City
Boulevard, Suite 1, Blacksburg, VA 24061.
Gary Skaggs, PhD, is Associate Professor, Department of Education Leadership
and Policy Studies at Virginia Tech.
Address correspondence to: Katherine M. Hertlein at the address above or (E-mail:
khertlein@yahoo.com).

The authors thank Jonathan Nevitt, PhD, and Lenore McWey, PhD, for their assis-
tance on this project. They also thank Gerhard Mels, PhD, of Scientific Software International for his help with the software.
This project was made possible by a grant from the Graduate School of Purdue University Calumet and the Graduate School of Purdue University.

[Haworth co-indexing entry note]: "Assessing the Relationship Between Differentiation and Infidelity: A
Structural Equation Model." Hertlein, Katherine M., and Gary Skaggs. Co-published simultaneously in *Journal of Couple & Relationship Therapy* (The Haworth Press) Vol. 4, No. 2/3, 2005, pp. 195-213; and: *Handbook of the Clinical Treatment of Infidelity* (ed: Fred P. Piercy, Katherine M. Hertlein, and Joseph L.
Wetchler) The Haworth Press, Inc., 2005, pp. 195-213. Single or multiple copies of this article are available
for a fee from The Haworth Document Delivery Service [1-800-HAWORTH, 9:00 a.m. - 5:00 p.m. (EST).
E-mail address: docdelivery@haworthpress.com].

Available online at http://www.haworthpress.com/web/JCRT
doi:10.1300/J398v04n02_16

plausible model of infidelity behavior, there are potentially other models that may be relevant in engaging in infidelity. The findings and implications are discussed. *[Article copies available for a fee from The Haworth Document Delivery Service: 1-800-HAWORTH. E-mail address: <docdelivery@haworthpress. com> Website: <http://www.HaworthPress.com> © 2005 by The Haworth Press, Inc. All rights reserved.]*

KEYWORDS. Differentiation, infidelity, two-step structural equation modeling, couples, anxiety management, causal models

INTRODUCTION

Infidelity has long been a concern for couples, families, and martial and family therapists (Atkins, Baucom, & Jacobson, 2001). Though a relationship with someone other than one's partner might manifest itself physically and/or emotionally, the bottom line is that the amount of shared time between one spouse and another individual outside of marriage becomes problematic for couples (Glass, personal communication, 2002). When time, energy, and resources are spent to maintain another relationship, the primary relationship is starved of attention, intimacy, and energy (Moultrup, 1990).

Though the incidence of extramarital relationships in our society changes from study to study, one aspect of these relationships remains stable: the impact created by extramarital infidelity can significantly damage relationships. In addition to the psychological impact of infidelity on both spouses (such as guilt, betrayal, loss of trust, loss of identity, and anger) additional physiological impacts exist such as stress, exhaustion, and chronic agitation (Spring, 1996). As a result, it is important for marital and family therapists to understand the processes in families and marriages where at least one partner has engaged in infidelity.

Several factors relate to infidelity. These factors include gender, education, age of individual, the duration of the primary relationship, level of religiosity, assessment of relationship satisfaction, and extramarital sexual permissiveness (Atkins, Baucom, & Jacobson, 2001; Buss & Shackelford, 1997; Oliver & Hyde, 1993; Treas & Giesen, 2000). The impact these factors have on infidelity, however, has been shown to differ from one study to another. More recent investigations have explored whether anxiety management may also be a factor in the likelihood of engaging in infidelity (Moultrup, 1990).

Differentiation, the term used to describe how one manages anxiety (Bowen, 1978), posits that one responds to anxiety through reacting in a patterned way (known as emotional process) or through making differentiated choices. In the present study, we sought to identify if factors related to differentiation are associated with one's likelihood of engaging in infidelity. We are adding to the previous literature on infidelity in several important ways. First, previous research seeking to predict variance in infidelity has used path diagrams (e.g., Reiss, Anderson, & Sponaugle, 1980); we present a structural equation model (SEM). SEM is not a method that is used often in the marital and family therapy literature. One advantage it has over other approaches is that it allows the researcher to incorporate information about the measurement properties of the instruments used. SEM also provides the researcher with a way to test whether the data are consistent with a theoretical approach.

Secondly, we select a measurement of infidelity behavior as a dependent variable as opposed to the more widely used measure of extramarital sexual permissiveness. In this way, we reduce any error associated with making an inferential jump between this attitudinal characteristic and actual behavior. Thirdly, this paper reflects an updated report of an infidelity model, since the most recent diagramming was published in the 1980s. Finally, the model in the present study incorporates differentiation into a model of infidelity, reducing focus on social background characteristics and increasing focusing on transgenerational factors.

DIFFERENTIATION AND INFIDELITY

Differentiation refers to one's ability to balance dependence and independence (Bowen, 1978; Friedman, 1991; Kerr & Bowen, 1988). Level of differentiation is reflective of one's ability to be involved in an intimate relationship and still remain independent. The more differentiated one is, the more likely individuality will be retained while in a group. Likewise, a less differentiated individual seeks approval from a group and clings for emotional support (Kerr & Bowen, 1988).

Differentiation and Anxiety Management

Differentiation describes how one manages anxiety (Bowen, 1978). Less differentiated people react to anxiety in an automatic and emotionally reactive manner; highly differentiated people are better able to monitor their emotional reactivity and have a greater capability of responding to challenging situations in a variety of ways. They do not react in an automatic fashion. Differentiation patterns in the family may be passed down through the generations and established in individuals at about the time they leave home or around the age of 21 (Bowen, 1978). Lawson, Gaushell, and Karst (1993), however, suggest differentiation might be established later in life, possibly not until the 4th or 5th decade.

Differentiation and Decision-Making

Differentiation is related to how one makes decisions in times of increased anxiety. One can make decisions based on engaging in patterned behavior or by exercising options and making different choices. Individuals with higher levels of differentiation are likely to explore options before emotionally reacting when they experience anxiety whereas persons with lower levels are likely to emotionally react, usually in their typical patterned behavior and are more likely to make decisions from a balanced perspective rather than emotional process.

In relation to sexual behavior, some view sexual acting out as a decision made rather than pathology (Levine, 1998). Connecting with differentiation as a decision-making process, individuals who engage in infidelity may not have explored options and may be emotionally reacting to anxiety experienced in their present relationship. Differentiation refers to decision-making and balance. It is this balance that may be central to understanding infidelity (Moultrup, 1990).

Differentiation, Anxiety, and Couples

Moultrup (1990) and Friedman (1991) have explicitly, but not empirically, tied differentiation and its supporting properties to infidelity. Friedman (1991) uses infidelity as a case example in which to apply Bowen systems theory. Moultrup (1990) contends that differentiation is "at the heart" of infidelity (p. 20). Because of differentiation's balance of dependence and independence, it makes sense that people who have difficulty balancing would pull away from their partners as a reaction, perhaps finding another partner, particularly if they are not particularly adept at maintaining independence while in a relationship.

In addition to tying the larger concept of differentiation to infidelity, Moultrup (1990) also identifies other properties of differentiation as they relate to infidelity. For example, Moultrup (1990) asserts that multigenerational patterns, fusion, triangulation, and emotional reactivity (all properties of differentiation), are related to infidelity. Individuals with familial patterns of engaging in infidelity might be more prone to engaging in infidelity when they experience periods of anxiety within their couple relationship. Additionally, others that typically have a pattern of involving other people in their problems as a way to reduce anxiety (triangulation) may do the same when they experience anxiety in their couple relationship, potentially increasing vulnerability to infidelity.

Milewski-Hertlein (2000) found after controlling for age and time, differentiation was related to infidelity. Specifically, women with higher levels of fusion and higher levels of emotional reactivity were more likely to engage in infidelity. Men with higher levels of individuation (i.e., defined as higher differentiation) were more likely to engage in infidelity. The differences in gender may be due to the difference in measuring differentiation (Milewski-Hertlein, 2000). As a result of these theoretical and research advancements in the area of understanding infidelity through a family systems lens, future research should continue the exploration of how differentiation is related to infidelity.

CAUSAL MODELS FOR UNDERSTANDING INFIDELITY

Infidelity has been a phenomenon that has been explored through a variety of statistical means. Path analyses have been used to determine the factors relating to extramarital sexual permissiveness (e.g., Reiss, Anderson, & Sponaugle, 1980). Research examining factors related to infidelity have focused on the previously mentioned factors, such as age, gender, and education. Little has been done in the way of developing causal relationships for understanding infidelity. Reiss, Anderson, and Sponaugle (1980), provide a model of understanding extramarital sexual permissiveness. This model serves as an early attempt to bring forth a causal explanation between social background variables and extramarital sexual permissiveness. The exogenous variables (causes) in the path analysis are education, gender, and age. The endogenous variables (effect) relating to extramarital sexual permissiveness are religiosity, gender equality, political liberty, marital happiness, and pre-marital sexual permissiveness. Overall, the model explains 17% of the variance in extramarital sexual permissiveness.

Saunders and Edwards (1984) build on the Reiss, Anderson, and Sponaugle (1980), path diagram by the addition of the variable "diffuse intimacy conception." In diffuse intimacy conception, a person places all of his or her energies into providing for one's partner and neglects personal needs (Reiss, Anderson, & Sponaugle, 1980; Saunders & Edwards, 1984). Individuals with diffuse intimacy conception experience difficulties sharing personal and private feelings with their partner, spending their energy focusing on meeting the perceived needs of their partner, not providing for their own needs (Saunders & Edwards, 1984). Saunders and Edwards (1984) argue that diffuse intimacy conception was theoretically related to marital satisfaction.

The exogenous variables in the Saunders and Edwards (1984) path diagram are age, gender, and education, the same as in the Reiss, Anderson, and Sponaugle model (1980). Saunders and Edwards (1984) construct separate paths for men and women. The full path diagram includes several variables: martial satisfaction, sexual satisfaction, priority of family roles, number of life stations, perceptions of power, diffuse intimacy conception, autonomy of heterosexual interaction, and comparison level of alternatives. The model explains 34% of the variance in extramarital sexual permissiveness for females and 16% of the variance for males. Edwards and Saunders (1984) conclude, ". . . the higher the level of diffuse intimacy conception, the more permissive the attitude toward extramarital sex" (p. 832).

Diffuse intimacy conception is related to differentiation in that diffuse intimacy conception refers to how one person meets his/her needs and their partner's needs in the relationship. In diffuse intimacy conception, one places energy into providing for their partner, but neglects their own needs (Reiss, Anderson, & Sponaugle, 1980; Saunders & Edwards, 1984). People with a diffuse intimacy conception experience difficulties sharing personal and private feelings with their partner. They also spend their energy focusing on meeting the perceived needs of their partner and not providing for their own needs (Saunders & Edwards, 1984). This relates to differentiation in that people with low levels of differentiation are likely to have their decisions influenced by others. Much of their energy is focused on putting forth towards their relationships, and spending energy seeking approval (Bowen, 1978).

THEORETICAL FRAMEWORK

Differentiation relates to how one responds to anxiety, either in an emotionally reactive manner, or in a manner reflecting greater options (Bowen, 1978). Differentiation is balancing independence and dependence in decisions when faced with anxiety. In the present study, differentiation is understood as being related to the decision to engage in infidelity. As individuals experience anxiety within their couple relationship, how do they handle it?

Individuals who are less differentiated are more emotionally reactive, more fused with others, might distance themselves from the relationship as a way to manage anxiety or use other methods (Bowen, 1978). In managing anxiety in these ways, individuals might be more prone to reacting to anxiety in their relationship by pulling in a third person. In some cases, this might mean engaging in infidelity.

METHOD

The present research adds to the existing knowledge base in several ways. First, this is the first path diagram using infidelity as the outcome variable instead of extramarital sexual permissiveness, an attitude. The present research presents a structural model exploring the manner in which anxiety manifests in one's relationships, adding onto the Saunders and Edwards (1984) model. Do factors related to differentiation impact one's likelihood of engaging in infidelity? The study provides a further step in using an existing infidelity scale and a scale measuring how one manages anxiety and how factors related to differentiation construct a model of infidelity. Finally, the present study can provide clinicians further variables to understand infidelity in a manner that will affect treatment. In this study, we predicted that Emotional Reactivity, Fusion with Parents, Distancing, and Ruminating (all anxiety-management methods that measure differentiation) would impact the likelihood of infidelity involvement.

Participants

A total of 119 students at a commuter campus voluntarily participated. The analysis included a total of 38 (31.9%) men and 81 (68.06%) women. Participant ages ranged from 18 to 53 years, with a mean age of 27.44 years. The total sample was composed of 8% African American,

2.4% Asian, 75.2% Caucasian, 12% Hispanic, and 1.6% identified themselves as "Other." Participants were required to be in a committed relationship for at least 6 months prior to the participation. Thirty-seven percent of the sample was married; 12% reported they were cohabitating; 46% reported they were dating. The mean duration of a relationship for the entire sample was 69.81 months (5.8175 years), with a range of 6 months to 31 years.

Measures

Differentiation of Self Inventory. The scale most appropriate for this study was the Differentiation of Self Inventory (DSI) developed by Skowron and Friedlander (1998). The DSI (Skowron & Friedlander, 1998) is a 43-item (six-point Likert) that included four subscales: Emotional Reactivity, I-Position, Emotional Cutoff, and Fusion with Others. The higher the score a participant receives on the scale, the higher level of differentiation. Emotional Reactivity is defined as the degree to which a person responds to his/her environment with too much emotion or hypersensitivity, and is composed of 11 items. Also composed of 11 items is the I-position scale. I-position refers to a clearly defined sense of self and an ability to adhere to what one believes even under pressure. Emotional Cutoff refers to an individual feeling threatened while in a close relationship with someone and feeling extremely vulnerable in the presence of others. There are a total of 12 items on this scale. Finally, Fusion with Others refers to when one is too emotionally involved with others, overidentified with parents, and/or triangulated (Skowron & Friedlander, 1998). This scale is composed of nine items.

Skowron and Friedlander (1998) report the DSI's reliability (Cronbach's alpha = .88) with good reliability for each of the subscales: Emotional Reactivity α = .84; I-Position α = .83; Emotional Cutoff α = .82; Fusion with others α = .74. Skowron and Friedlander (1998) developed the Differentiation of Self Inventory (DSI) through several levels of factor analyses. First, Skowron and Friedlander (1998) performed a principal components analysis followed by an orthogonal rotation, resulting in four factors with eigenvalues over one. The items associated with these four factors were then revised to better adhere to theory, and tested again. After low item-scale correlations, another 35 items were not included, leaving 43 items on the DSI.

Infidelity Scale. The Infidelity Scale, presented by Drigotas, Safstrom, and Gentilia (1999), measures physical and emotional infidelity by assessing the intensity of a relationship with someone to whom the respondent is attracted other than the person's partner. Drigotas, Safstrom, and Gentilia (1999) determined there were three types of infidelity measured by the scale–Physical Infidelity, Emotional Infidelity, and Composite Infidelity. The Physical Infidelity subscale consisted of six items, and Cronbach's alpha level for this subscale is .83. A sample item is "How much physical contact have you had with this other person?" Five items made up the Emotional infidelity scale, with Cronbach's alpha level of .84. This scale measures the emotional connection that one has to another person, with a sample item of "How much time did you spend thinking about this other person?" The composite infidelity variable was identified through a factor analysis, where 9 of the 11 items loaded on a factor Drigotas, Safstrom, and Gentilia (1999) termed Composite Infidelity. Sample items include "How much time did you spend with this other person?" and "How physically intimate were you with this person?" (p. 523).

Procedures

The researchers solicited participants from classes at a Midwest commuter college campus. Each participant completed the Differentiation of Self Inventory (Skowron & Friedlander, 1998). Participants also completed the Infidelity scale developed by Drigotas, Safstrom, and Gentilia (1999). The survey was administered during classes.

Data Analysis

Data were initially analyzed through exploratory factor analyses. After the factor analyses, a structural model was created to determine the relationship between the differentiation factors (Emotional Reactivity, Fusion with Parents, Distancing, Rumination, and Physical and Emotional Infidelity). Latent variable modeling is an appropriate practice for variables related to counseling (Fassinger, 1987). A two-step structural equation modeling procedure was used (Anderson & Gerbing, 1988; Bollen, 1989; Schumacker & Lomax, 1996).

RESULTS

Exploratory Factor Analysis for DSI

There were two reasons we performed a new exploratory factor analysis. First, as factor analysis is data driven and we were using a different sample than the original study, it was appropriate to rerun the factor analysis. Secondly, we believed that the factors were correlated and thus, felt it appropriate to run an oblique rotation as opposed an orthogonal rotation, which was used in the original study. We used SPSS version 11.0 (SPSS, 2002) and initially performed a principal components analysis with an oblique rotation with Kaiser Normalization. After the exploratory factory analysis on the differentiation subscale, 17 of the original 43 items loaded onto the factors. The number of factors was set to four to determine if the results of the new EFA was similar to the original subscales. Items were loaded onto factors if their pattern matrix coefficient was above .50.

Based on the exploratory factor analysis, the factors for each scale in the present study were different than in the initial validation of the instrument. The four subscales from the Differentiation of Self Inventory became: Emotional Reactivity, Fusion with Parents, Distancing, and Ruminating. Though Skowron and Friedlander (1998) also had a factor called "Emotional Reactivity," the remaining three subscales seemed to have different meaning from the original subscales. A likely reason for this is that factor analysis is data-driven. Since the sample used in the present study was different from a sample used in the previous studies, a sample difference may have resulted in the different factor loadings and different categories.

The present Emotional Reactivity factor was composed of five items. Its items assess how reactive respondents perceive themselves to be. Three of the items were recoded; higher scores on the scale mean higher levels of differentiation. The alpha coefficient for the Emotional Reactivity scale was .73.

The Fusion with Parents factor was composed of four items. One item was recoded because, again, higher scores on the scale refer to higher levels of differentiation. The alpha coefficient for this scale was .79. The Fusion with Parents subscale refers to the respondent's level of emotional attachment. It differs from the Fusion with Others subscale in the original DSI validation study (Skowron & Friedlander, 1998) in that the items on the Fusion with Parents subscale refer to level of involvement with the respondent's parents and family members, whereas the items on the Fusion with Others subscale refers to the respondent's level of emotional involvement with others, but includes parents.

The Distancing factor was composed of items assessing the distance one puts in between themselves and others in times of stress or anxiety. It was composed of five items. All items were recoded, again, to reflect that higher scores on the scale refer to higher levels of differentiation. The alpha coefficient was .71.

Finally, the Ruminating factor was composed of three items. The items appeared to have elements of how long one persists in thinking about anxiety and other negative feelings. All items were also recoded on this scale, and the alpha coefficient was .54. Means and standard deviations of the subscales can be found in Table 1.

The four factors–Emotional Reactivity, Fusion with Parents, Distancing, and Rumination–were the variables used to measure differentiation and how one manages anxiety. First, Emotional Reactivity is a concept that Bowen (1978) discusses in relation to differentiation and managing anxiety. Those individuals with lower levels of differentiation are more like to emotionally react rather than exercising options and alternatives. Secondly, those who are more fused with their family and others cling to a group before feeling comfortable to make their own decisions (Bowen, 1978). Individuals with higher levels of fusion have lower levels of differentiation and respond to anxiety through reacting as opposed to generating options of their own. Third, Distancing is related to both differentiation and infidelity. Those who experience anxiety in relationships and have lower levels of differentiation deal with anxiety through distancing themselves from the partners and their problems, resulting in Intimacy Avoidant affairs (Brown, 1991). Finally, Ruminating refers to anxiety management and differentiation because an individual who has a difficult time managing anxiety may be more

TABLE 1. Means and Standard Deviations on the Modified DSI and Infidelity Scale

Scale	Total	
	Mean	*SD*
Emotional Reactivity	19.807	4.132
Fusion with Parents	14.277	3.757
Distancing	21.723	5.140
Ruminating	10.202	3.50
Physical Infidelity	15.057	9.384
Temptation Infidelity	18.916	8.283

prone to think about the event all day. This could in fact be an emotionally reactive pattern.

Exploratory Factor Analysis for Infidelity Scale

The exploratory factor analysis for the Infidelity scale was performed in the same manner as for the Differentiation of Self Inventory. Again, an oblique rotation was used because the factors are likely to correlate with one another. Two factors emerged–one factor relating to Physical Infidelity and another relating to items assessing temptation to engage in infidelity, called Temptation Infidelity.

The scale with items relating to Physical Infidelity was different than in the original factor analysis performed for the Infidelity Scales. Four items from the original Infidelity Scale (Drigotas, Safstrom, & Gentilia, 1999) loaded on the Physical Infidelity factor. Four items loaded on the Temptation Infidelity scale. The alpha coefficients for the Physical Infidelity subscale and Temptation Infidelity were .87 and .85, respectively. Means and standard deviations for the modified Infidelity scale (with the factors Physical and Temptation Infidelity) are presented in Table 1. Table 2 presents the correlation matrix of the four subscales of differentiation and the two subscales of the Infidelity Scale.

Two-Step Structural Equation Modeling

We employed a two-step structural equation modeling procedure (Anderson & Gerbing, 1988; Schumaker & Lomax, 1996). There are

TABLE 2. Correlation Matrix of Differentiation and Infidelity Subscales

Subscales	1	2	3	4	5	6
1. Emotional Reactivity	1.00	.198*	.087	.265*	−.089	−.129
2. Fusion with Parents		1.00	.152	−.170	.139	.120
3. Distancing			1.00	−.015	−.179	−.069
4. Ruminating				1.00	−.122	−.109
5. Temptation Infidelity					1.00	.705*
6. Physical Infidelity						1.00

* = $p < .05$

several advantages of a two-step structural modeling approach (Anderson & Gerbing, 1988). One advantage is that the researcher can test the measurement models both pre- and post-modification indices prior to working with the structural model. Researchers employing a two-step modeling procedures can also make better causal inferences. Another advantage is the separate assessment of the measurement models and the structural model. This means that the researcher can determine whether the goodness-of-fit of the measurement model influences into the structural model (Anderson & Gebring, 1988).

In the present study, we assessed the measurement models for the 25 observed variables (the 17 items on the Differentiation of Self inventory and the eight items on the Infidelity Scale) and the six latent variables (Emotional Reactivity, Fusion with Parents, Distancing, Ruminating, Physical Infidelity, and Temptation Infidelity). The initial measurement model was significant, p < .001 (see Table 3 for goodness-of-fit estimates). The good fit of the measurement models was not surprising, given the results of the exploratory factor analysis. What we are interested in was the structural model–what is the relationship between these variables while considering their measurement properties?

The next step in the measurement phase was to make appropriate alterations as indicated by the modification indices provided in the LISREL output. After the theoretically appropriate modification indices were made, the final measurement model was analyzed and was found to have good fit (see Table 3). Figure 1 shows the measurement models in the present study.

The final step in the two-step structural equation modeling procedure was to impose the structural model on the measurement models. The results showed that the Comparative Fit Index (CFI) was above .90, indicating the model was a good fit (Schumacker & Lomax, 1996) (see Table 3.).

For the sample in this study, Emotional Reactivity, Fusion with Parents, Distancing, and Rumination were not related to Physical Infidelity or Temptation Infidelity. In other words, those with lower levels of Emotional Reactivity, Fusion with Parents, Distancing, and Rumination were not more or less likely to engage in infidelity. This model, however, is inconsistent in its goodness-of-fit estimates. For example, the Normed Fit Index (NFI) was lower than the Comparative Fit Index (CFI). In a model that represents good fit, both of these numbers would be close to one (Raykov & Marcoulides, 2000). This means that the model presented is a plausible model, but that there are other models that may be just as plausible or better (Schumacker & Lomax, 1996).

TABLE 3. Summary of Model-Fit Statistics

Model	χ^2	df	p-value	NFI	NNFI	CFI	GFI	AGFI
Initial CFA	431.58	260	< .001	.70	.83	.85	.79	.73
Final CFA	340.70	254	< .001	.76	.91	.92	.81	.76
Structural Model	350.49	260	< .001	.76	.91	.92	.81	.76

FIGURE 1. This figure presents the measurement models for differentiation and infidelity subscales in the present study. These models were generated via confirmatory factor analysis.

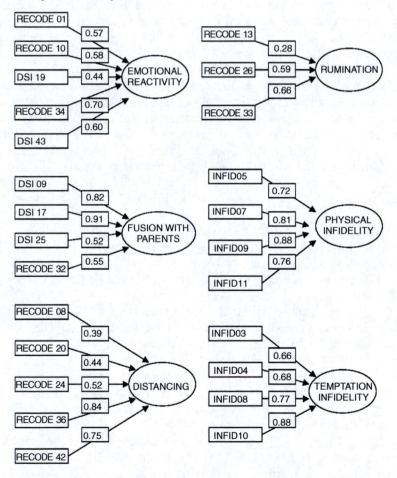

After the standardized solution was obtained (see Figure 2), it was apparent that the differentiation factors of Emotional Reactivity, Fusion with Parents, Distancing, and Rumination, were not strongly related to engaging in Physical Infidelity or the Temptation Infidelity Scale. The standardized regression coefficients for Emotional Reactivity, Fusion with Parents, Distancing, and Rumination to Physical Infidelity were $-.15$, $.08$, $-.14$ and $.04$, respectively. The regression coefficients for the factors related to Temptation Infidelity was $.04$ for Emotional Reactivity, $.00$ for Fusion with Parents, and $.10$ for Distancing. Rumination was not included in the model toward Temptation Infidelity because, unlike the other variables that have been related to infidelity in previous literature, the Rumination factor had no support in the literature for relating it to Temptation Infidelity. There are no indirect effects for Physical Infidelity because there was no path from Temptation Infidelity to Physical Infidelity. This decision was made because individuals who are tempted to engage in infidelity do not necessarily engage in infidelity. See Table 4 for direct effects, indirect effects, and total effects. Additionally, there was no path from Temptation infidelity to Distancing or Ruminating, as there was no literature in the field indicating a path would make sense.

FIGURE 2. This figure presents the structural model for the relationship between differentiation and infidelity (standardized solution)

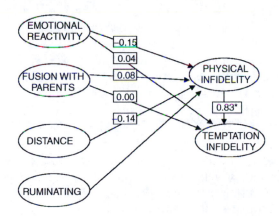

* = p < .05

TABLE 4. Direct, Indirect, and Total Effects of Independent Variables on Infidelity

Variables	Direct Effects on Temptation Infidelity	Indirect Effect on Temptation Infidelity	Total Effects on Temptation Infidelity	Direct Effects on Physical Infidelity	Total Effects on Physical Infidelity
Emotional Reactivity	.04	−.09	−.05	−.15	−.15
Fusion with Parents	.00	.06	.06	.08	.08
Distancing	−.10	−.10	−.20	−.14	−.14
Ruminating	0.0	0.0	0.0	0.4	0.4
Physical Infidelity	.83	--	.83	--	--

DISCUSSION

The factor analyses in the present study were consistent with theory. The exploratory factor analysis of the DSI revealed that 17 variables loaded on four factors–Emotional Reactivity, Fusion with Parents, Distancing, and Ruminating. Support for these factors come from Bowen's theory of differentiation. Additionally, two factors emerged from the exploratory factor analysis from the Infidelity Scale, related to physical involvement in infidelity and being tempted to engage in infidelity. The results in this study indicated that Emotional Reactivity, Fusion with Parents, Distancing, and Rumination may not be related to infidelity. This result contrasts other research (Milewski-Hertlein, 2000), relating fusion, emotional reactivity, and other properties of differentiation to infidelity. Structural equation modeling provides a correction for attenuation. In other words, it provides an analysis of a relationship between two or more latent factors while correcting for the measurement error. Once controlling for measurement error, there was no demonstrated relationship between differentiation factors and infidelity.

The results of this study might be due to several factors. First, the sample in this study was different from the sample in the Skowron and Friedlander (1998) initial validation study of the Differentiation of Self Inventory (DSI). In the initial validation of the study, students and faculty from a university participated (Skowron & Friedlander, 1998). In the present study, students from a commuter campus were used. Since factor analysis is data driven, it is quite possible that differences in population would yield different results. We also used a different number of items from the original DSI-17 of the original 43. This also might account for the differences in results. One further explanation might be the different powers of the statistical tests used. The more powerful the test, such as SEM, the more difficult it will be to prove that there is a difference.

Secondly, age of the respondents might also be a factor for the inconsistency in results. The sample in the present study had a mean of 27.44 years. As far as differentiation, Lawson, Gaushell, and Karst (1993), in contrast to Bowen, posit that one's level of differentiation is not secure until later in life, well beyond an individual's 20s. Given this information, the participants in the present study would not have a stable level of differentiation, according to Lawson, Gaushell, and Karst (1993).

The age of the present sample might also impact the results within the infidelity variables. This study might have more weight with older respondents as younger individuals may have relationships more in flux. Additionally, Atkins, Baucom, and Jacobson (2001) indicate that men between 55-65 are more likely to engage in infidelity, and women between the ages of 40-45 are more likely to engage in infidelity. As a result, the group in their twenties that has no reported infidelity might engage in infidelity at a later point in their lives. The present study did not account for accumulative incidence of infidelity (Thompson, 1983).

Limitations

One limitation might be the measurement of differentiation and infidelity. Concepts such as Emotional Reactivity, Fusion with Parents, and other concepts related to differentiation are difficult to measure with a pencil and paper inventory. Another limitation of the DSI specifically might be the type of differentiation measured. There are two types of differentiation–basic and functional. Basic differentiation refers to one's general level of differentiation that they acquire from one's family of origin, stable over time (Bowen, 1978). As events occur in one's life, the functional level of differentiation changes. Physical infidelity, like any other behavior, may be an event. In the DSI, it may be likely that one's basic level of differentiation is being measured and compared with infidelity, which is an event and more reflective of functional differentiation. Finally, no other variables such as age, duration of relationship, or gender were included in the analyses. Another model incorporating all of these, specifically one model accounting for gender, might increase model fit.

Implications

Though the results in the present study are inconclusive as to the extent that Emotional Reactivity, Fusion with Parents, Distancing, and

Rumination are related to infidelity, there are several implications for therapists, theorists, and family therapy researchers. Therapists can use this information to examine in what other ways anxiety management in individuals does or does not contribute to engaging in infidelity. Theorists can continue to explore transgenerational variables such as emotional reactivity, fusion with parents, and other factors to identify what comprises decision-making in reaction to anxiety within a couple. Finally, researchers can work to build better measurement tools for examining these abstract concepts.

Future Research

Future research might inspire clinicians to generate better measurement tools for such concepts as Emotional Reactivity, Fusion with Parents, Distancing, and other components related to differentiation. The present study could also be conducted with a larger sample and different population, as well as the inclusion of other variables that may be related to infidelity.

NOTE

1. Hu and Bentler (1999) report that cutoff value "close" to .95 for Maximum Likelihood-based CFI indicates a good fit between model and data, as it appears to result in less Type II error rates. However, they also recommend researchers use a combination of measures to assess model fit, such as consideration of the RMSEA.

REFERENCES

Anderson, J. C., & Gerbing, D. W. (1988). Structural equation modeling in practice: A review and recommended two-step approach. *Psychological Bulletin, 103*(3), 411-423.

Atkins, D. C., Baucom, D. H., & Jacobson, N. S. (2001). Understanding infidelity: Correlates in a national random sample. *Journal of Family Psychology, 15*(4), 735-749.

Bollen, K. A. (1989). Structural equations with latent variables. New York, NY: John Wiley & Sons.

Bowen, M. (1978). *Family therapy in clinical practice.* Northvale, NJ: Aronson.

Buss, D. M., & Shackelford, T. K. (1997). Susceptibility to infidelity in the first year of marriage. *Journal of Research in Personality, 31*,193-221.

Crocker, L., & Algina, J. (1986). Introduction to classical and modern test theory. Orlando, FL: Harcourt, Brace, & Jovanovich.

Drigotas, S. M., Safstrom, C. A., & Gentilia, T. (1999). An investment model prediction of dating infidelity. *Journal of Personality & Social Psychology, 77*(3), 509-524.

Fassinger, R. E. (1987). Use of structural equation modeling in counseling psychology research. *Journal of Counseling Psychology, 34*(4), 425-436.

Friedman, E. H. (1991). Bowen theory and therapy. In A. S. Gurman & D. P. Kniskern (Eds.), *Handbook of Family Therapy* (Vol. 2, pp. 134-170). Bristol, PA: Brunner/Mazel.

Hu, L., & Bentler, P. M. (1999). Cutoff criteria for fit indexes in covariance structure analysis: Conventional criteria versus new alternatives. *Structural Equation Modeling, 6*(1), 1-55.

Jöreskog, K., & Sörbom, D. (1996). *LISREL 8: User's reference guide.* Chicago, IL: Scientific Software International.

Kerr, M. E., & Bowen, M. (1988). *Family evaluation.* New York, NY: W. W. Norton & Company.

Lawson, D., Gaushell, H., & Karst, R. (1993). The age of personal authority in the family system. *Journal of Marital & Family Therapy, 19*(3), 287-292.

Levine, S. B. (1998). Extramarital sexual affairs. *Journal of Sex & Marital Therapy, 24*(3), 207-216.

Milewski-Hertlein, K. (2000). *The role of differentiation and triangulation in extradyadic relationships.* Unpublished master's thesis, Purdue University Calumet.

Moultrup, D. J. (1990). *Husbands, wives, and lovers: The emotional system of the extramarital affair.* New York: The Guilford Press.

Raykov, T., & Marcoulides, G. A. (2000). *A first course in structural equation modeling.* Mahwah, NJ: Lawrence Elbaum Associates.

Reiss, I. L., Anderson, R. E., & Sponaugle, G. C. (1980). A multivariate model of the determinants of extramarital sexual permissiveness. *Journal of Marriage and the Family, 42*(2), 395-411.

Saunders, J. M., & Edwards, J. N. (1984). Extramarital sexuality: A predictive model of permissive attitudes. *Journal of Marriage and the Family, 46*(4), 825-835.

Schumacker, R. E., & Lomax, R. G. (1996). *A beginner's guide to structural equation modeling.* Mahwah, NJ: Lawrence Elbaum Associates.

Skowron, E. A., & Friedlander, M. L. (1998). The Differentiation of Self Inventory: Development and initial validation. *Journal of Counseling Psychology, 45*(3), 235-246.

Spring, J. A. (1996). *After the affair: Healing the pain and rebuilding the trust when a partner has been unfaithful.* New York, NY: Harper Collins.

SPSS (2002). Chicago, IL: SPSS Inc.

Thompson, A. P. (1983). Extramarital sex: A review of the research literature. *Journal of Sex Research, 19*(1), 1-22.

Treas, J., & Giesen, D. (2000). Sexual infidelity among married and cohabitating Americans. *Journal of Marriage and the Family, 62,* 48-60.

Index

Accessibility, Internet infidelity and, 10

Accidental infidelity, 120

Accusatory suffering, 2
   case example of, 87-90
   defined, 84-86
   therapist's options for, 86-87

Addiction, Internet, 124

Affairs, 136. *See also* Infidelity; Split Self Affairs
   cultural myths about, 2
   defined, 9
   mathematics of frequency of, 162-164
   myths about, 162-164
   myths about what people are searching for and, 164-166
   nonsense about, 2
   problem of underlying dynamic in, 167-170
   thinking clearly about, 170-171
   what they're really about, 167-170

Affordability, Internet infidelity and, 10

Anonymity, Internet infidelity and, 10

Anonymous sexual encounters, 151

Anxiety management, differentiation and, 198

Anxiety, Internet relationships and, 123

Apology, 42-43,96-97
   process of, 49-53
   role of, 2

Attachment injuries, 23-28,94

Attachment theory, 19-21

Atwood, Joan, 2

Bettinger, Michael, 3

Blow, Adrian, 2

Bollas, Christopher, 114

Bonds, emotional, 20-21

Boundaries, 159

Bowen systems theory, 13

Brown, Emily, 3

Carr, Adrian, 2

Case, Brian, 2

Clinical practices, recommendations for, 189-192

Collaboration, Internet infidelity and, 10

Communication
   building, treating Internet infidelity and, 128-129
   Internet infidelity and, 10,123-124

Communities online, Internet infidelity and, 10

Countertransference, 152-155

Couples therapy, for Split Self Affairs, 58-60

Couples, effects of infidelity on, 7-8

Crisis intervention, treating Internet infidelity and, 126,141-142

Cyber affairs. *See* Internet infidelity

Cyber infidelity. *See* Internet infidelity

Cyber-Affairs, 120-121

Cyber-cheating, 104-105

Cyber-flirting, 107

Cyber-Flirts, 119-120

Cyber-lovers, loss of, 127-128

Cyber-sex, 120

Cyberspace. *See also* Internet